FEEDING AND EATING DISORDERS

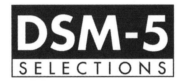

FEEDING AND EATING DISORDERS

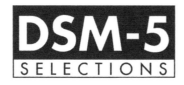

American Psychiatric Association

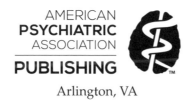

AMERICAN
PSYCHIATRIC
ASSOCIATION
PUBLISHING

Arlington, VA

Manufactured in the United States of America on acid-free paper.

ISBN 978-1-61537-012-2 (Paperback)

American Psychiatric Association
1000 Wilson Boulevard
Arlington, VA 22209-3901
www.psych.org

Feeding and Eating Disorders: DSM-5® Selections is an anthology published by the American Psychiatric Association from the following sources:

American Psychiatric Association: *Diagnostic and Statistical Manual of Mental Disorders*, Fifth Edition. Arlington, VA, American Psychiatric Association, 2013

Black, DW; Grant, JE: *DSM-5® Guidebook: The Essential Companion to the Diagnostic and Statistical Manual of Mental Disorders, Fifth Edition.* Washington, DC, American Psychiatric Publishing, 2014

Barnhill JW: *DSM-5® Clinical Cases.* Washington, DC, American Psychiatric Publishing, 2014

Muskin, PR: *DSM-5® Self-Exam Questions: Test Questions for the Diagnostic Criteria.* Washington, DC, American Psychiatric Publishing, 2014

Contents

Introduction to DSM-5® Selections

Welcome to *DSM-5 Selections*. The purpose of this series is to educate readers about important diagnostic issues associated with categories of DSM-5 disorders. The initial books in the ***DSM-5 Selections*** series are *Sleep-Wake Disorders, Depressive Disorders, Schizophrenia Spectrum and Other Psychotic Disorders, Feeding and Eating Disorders, Neurodevelopmental Disorders,* and *Anxiety Disorders.* Each book in the series includes the diagnostic criteria relevant to the disorders included in each category. The criteria are taken directly from DSM-5, the most comprehensive, current, and critical resource for clinical practice available today. Also included in each book in the series are extracts from the ***DSM-5 Guidebook, DSM-5 Clinical Cases,*** and ***DSM-5 Self-Exam Questions.*** Consequently, each book in the series offers readers a unique introduction to individual categories of DSM-5 disorders and an opportunity to test one's knowledge about DSM-5 disorders.

DSM-5 Guidebook serves as a roadmap to DSM-5 disorders for clinicians and researchers. It illuminates the content of DSM-5 by teaching mental health professionals how to use the revised diagnostic criteria, and it provides practical content for its clinical use. The book offers a fresh perspective to DSM diagnostic categories by focusing on the changes between DSM-IV-TR and DSM-5 that will most significantly impact clinical application of the criteria.

DSM-5 Clinical Cases presents composite patient cases that exemplify the diagnostic criteria for disorders contained in a category. ***DSM-5 Clinical Cases*** makes DSM-5 come alive for teachers, students, and clinicians. The book helps readers to understand diagnostic concepts, including symptoms, severity, comorbidities, age of onset and development, dimensionality across disorders, and gender and cultural implications.

The questions in ***DSM-5 Self-Exam Questions*** were written to test readers' knowledge of conceptual changes to DSM-5, specific changes to diagnoses, and the diagnostic criteria. Each question includes short answers that explain the rationale for each correct answer and contain important information on diagnostic classification, criteria sets, diagnoses, codes, severity, culture, age, and gender. The questions are helpful for preparing for various examinations.

The ***DSM-5 Selections*** series is not intended to replace DSM-5 or the other books from which the extracts are taken. Rather, the series is intended to give readers key selected materials that pertain directly to specific disorder categories. If you find that you require more information about a specific disorder or category of disorders, you are encouraged to examine an APP textbook or clinical manual. You can review the full list of APP titles at www.appi.org.

Robert E. Hales, M.D.
Editor-in-Chief

Preface

There are eight feeding and eating disorders described in DSM-5. Three of these occur in childhood: pica, rumination disorder, and avoidant/restrictive food intake disorder. The relative prevalence of these disorders and the risk factors are not readily apparent. Three major disorders that occur in adolescence or adulthood are anorexia nervosa, bulimia nervosa, and binge-eating disorder.

Anorexia nervosa is a severe psychiatric disorder that affects women at a rate of approximately 0.4% point prevalence. The long-term mortality from anorexia nervosa is the highest of any psychiatric disorder. Most common causes of mortality are suicide and multiorgan system failure. Bulimia nervosa is more common than anorexia nervosa in adults, with a point prevalence of approximately 2% of women.

Finally, binge-eating disorder, a new DSM-5 diagnosis, is reported to have a prevalence rate of 3.5% among women and 2% among men. Although the highest rates of all three disorders are in adolescence, adults may also develop these disorders.

Psychiatric comorbidity occurs frequently in all of the eating disorders. The most frequent comorbid condition in patients with anorexia nervosa is major depressive disorder. The diagnosis of depressive disorders is problematic and is compounded by the fact that low body weight frequently results in mood changes. Anxiety disorders are also commonly seen in anorexia nervosa, and higher-than-expected rates of substance use disorders are frequently reported.

Similar to patients with anorexia nervosa, patients with bulimia nervosa have high rates of mood disorders, especially major depression. Suicidality is also higher than expected in this population. It is important to note that there is a high rate of posttraumatic stress disorder (37%) in patients who have been diagnosed with bulimia nervosa. The patients also have high rates of substance use disorder.

With regard to binge-eating disorder, patients are at high rates of other co-occurring psychiatric disorders. Approximately 20%–25% of individuals with binge-eating disorder also have significant substance use disorders, similar to individuals with bulimia nervosa and anorexia nervosa. The most common comorbid psychiatric disorder is depression, which affects about 50% of individuals with binge-eating disorder. Finally, there are reasonably high rates of anxiety disorders, particularly panic disorder and simple phobia.

In summary, anorexia nervosa and bulimia nervosa have relatively high rates of mortality, and comorbid medical complications are common. Consequently, clinicians should be knowledgeable about both these conditions and others contained within the category of feeding and eating disorders.

Adapted with permission from Mitchell JE, Wonderlich SA: "Feeding and Eating Disorders," in *The American Psychiatric Publishing Textbook of Psychiatry*, 6th Edition. Edited by Hales RE, Yudofsky SC, Roberts LW. Washington, DC, American Psychiatric Publishing, 2014, pp. 557–586.

The changes made to the DSM-5 diagnostic criteria for feeding and eating disorders are highlighted below. This is not meant to be an exhaustive guide to DSM-5 changes, and minor changes in text or wording made for clarity are not described. Section I of DSM-5 contains a full description of changes pertaining to the chapter organization in DSM-5, the multiaxial system, and the introduction of dimensional assessments.

Highlights of Changes From DSM-IV-TR to DSM-5

In DSM-5, the feeding and eating disorders include several disorders included in DSM-IV as *feeding and eating disorders of infancy or early childhood* in the chapter "Disorders Usually First Diagnosed in Infancy, Childhood, or Adolescence." In addition, brief descriptions and preliminary diagnostic criteria are provided for several conditions under *other specified feeding and eating disorder;* information about these conditions is currently insufficient to document their clinical characteristics and validity or to provide definitive diagnostic criteria.

Pica and Rumination Disorder

The DSM-IV criteria for pica and for rumination disorder have been revised for clarity and to indicate that the diagnoses can be made for individuals of any age.

Avoidant/Restrictive Food Intake Disorder

DSM-IV feeding disorder of infancy or early childhood has been renamed avoidant/restrictive food intake disorder, and the criteria have been significantly expanded. The DSM-IV disorder was rarely used, and limited information is available on the characteristics, course, and outcome of this disorder. Additionally, a large number of individuals, primarily but not exclusively children and adolescents, substantially restrict their food intake and experience significant associated physiological or psychosocial problems, but their presentation does not meet criteria for any DSM-IV eating disorder. Avoidant/restrictive food intake disorder is a broad category intended to capture this range of presentations.

Anorexia Nervosa

The core diagnostic criteria for anorexia nervosa are conceptually unchanged from DSM-IV with one exception: the requirement for amenorrhea has been eliminated. In DSM-IV, this requirement was waived in a number of situations (e.g., for males, for females taking contraceptives). In addition, the clinical characteristics and course of females meeting all DSM-IV criteria for anorexia nervosa except amenorrhea closely resemble those of females meeting all DSM-IV criteria. As in DSM-IV, individuals with this disorder are required by Criterion A to be at a significantly low body weight for their developmental stage. The wording of the criterion has been changed for clarity, and guidance regarding how to judge whether an individual is at or below a significantly low weight is now provided in the text. Criterion B has been expanded, in

DSM-5, to include not only overtly expressed fear of weight gain but also persistent behavior that interferes with weight gain.

Bulimia Nervosa

The only change to the DSM-IV criteria for bulimia nervosa is a reduction in the required minimum average frequency of binge eating and inappropriate compensatory behavior frequency from twice to once weekly. The clinical characteristics and outcome of individuals meeting this slightly lower threshold are similar to those meeting the DSM-IV criterion.

Binge-Eating Disorder

Extensive research followed the promulgation of preliminary criteria for binge-eating disorder in Appendix B of DSM-IV, and findings supported the clinical utility and validity of binge-eating disorder. The only significant difference from the preliminary DSM-IV criteria is that the minimum average frequency of binge eating required for diagnosis has been changed from at least twice weekly for 6 months to at least once weekly over the last 3 months, which is identical to the DSM-5 frequency criterion for bulimia nervosa.

Elimination Disorders

No significant changes have been made to the elimination disorders diagnostic class from DSM-IV to DSM-5. The disorders in this chapter were previously classified under *disorders usually first diagnosed in infancy, childhood, or adolescence* in DSM-IV and exist now as an independent classification in DSM-5.

DSM-5® Feeding and Eating Disorders: ICD-9-CM and ICD-10-CM Codes

Disorder	ICD-9-CM	ICD-10-CM
Pica	307.52	
In children		F98.3
In adults		F50.8
Rumination Disorder	307.53	F98.21
Avoidant/Restrictive Food Intake Disorder	307.59	F50.8
Anorexia Nervosa	307.1	
Restricting type		F50.01
Binge-eating/purging type		F50.02
Bulimia Nervosa	307.51	F50.2
Binge-Eating Disorder	307.51	F50.8
Other Specified Feeding or Eating Disorder	307.59	F50.8
Unspecified Feeding or Eating Disorder	307.50	F50.9

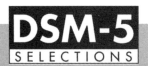

Feeding and Eating Disorders
Diagnostic and Statistical Manual of Mental Disorders, Fifth Edition

Feeding and eating disorders are characterized by a persistent disturbance of eating or eating-related behavior that results in the altered consumption or absorption of food and that significantly impairs physical health or psychosocial functioning. Diagnostic criteria are provided for pica, rumination disorder, avoidant/restrictive food intake disorder, anorexia nervosa, bulimia nervosa, and binge-eating disorder.

The diagnostic criteria for rumination disorder, avoidant/restrictive food intake disorder, anorexia nervosa, bulimia nervosa, and binge-eating disorder result in a classification scheme that is mutually exclusive, so that during a single episode, only one of these diagnoses can be assigned. The rationale for this approach is that, despite a number of common psychological and behavioral features, the disorders differ substantially in clinical course, outcome, and treatment needs. A diagnosis of pica, however, may be assigned in the presence of any other feeding and eating disorder.

Some individuals with disorders described in this chapter report eating-related symptoms resembling those typically endorsed by individuals with substance use disorders, such as craving and patterns of compulsive use. This resemblance may reflect the involvement of the same neural systems, including those implicated in regulatory self-control and reward, in both groups of disorders. However, the relative contributions of shared and distinct factors in the development and perpetuation of eating and substance use disorders remain insufficiently understood.

Finally, obesity is not included in DSM-5 as a mental disorder. Obesity (excess body fat) results from the long-term excess of energy intake relative to energy expenditure. A range of genetic, physiological, behavioral, and environmental factors that vary across individuals contributes to the development of obesity; thus, obesity is not considered a mental disorder. However, there are robust associations between obesity and a number of mental disorders (e.g., binge-eating disorder, depressive and bipolar disorders, schizophrenia). The side effects of some psychotropic medications contribute importantly to the development of obesity, and obesity may be a risk factor for the development of some mental disorders (e.g., depressive disorders).

Pica

Diagnostic Criteria

A. Persistent eating of nonnutritive, nonfood substances over a period of at least 1 month.
B. The eating of nonnutritive, nonfood substances is inappropriate to the developmental level of the individual.

C. The eating behavior is not part of a culturally supported or socially normative practice.

D. If the eating behavior occurs in the context of another mental disorder (e.g., intellectual disability [intellectual developmental disorder], autism spectrum disorder, schizophrenia) or medical condition (including pregnancy), it is sufficiently severe to warrant additional clinical attention.

Coding note: The ICD-9-CM code for pica is **307.52** and is used for children or adults. The ICD-10-CM codes for pica are **(F98.3)** in children and **(F50.8)** in adults.

Specify if:

   In remission: After full criteria for pica were previously met, the criteria have not been met for a sustained period of time.

Diagnostic Features

The essential feature of pica is the eating of one or more nonnutritive, nonfood substances on a persistent basis over a period of at least 1 month (Criterion A) that is severe enough to warrant clinical attention. Typical substances ingested tend to vary with age and availability and might include paper, soap, cloth, hair, string, wool, soil, chalk, talcum powder, paint, gum, metal, pebbles, charcoal or coal, ash, clay, starch, or ice. The term *nonfood* is included because the diagnosis of pica does not apply to ingestion of diet products that have minimal nutritional content. There is typically no aversion to food in general. The eating of nonnutritive, nonfood substances must be developmentally inappropriate (Criterion B) and not part of a culturally supported or socially normative practice (Criterion C). A minimum age of 2 years is suggested for a pica diagnosis to exclude developmentally normal mouthing of objects by infants that results in ingestion. The eating of nonnutritive, nonfood substances can be an associated feature of other mental disorders (e.g., intellectual disability [intellectual developmental disorder], autism spectrum disorder, schizophrenia). If the eating behavior occurs exclusively in the context of another mental disorder, a separate diagnosis of pica should be made only if the eating behavior is sufficiently severe to warrant additional clinical attention (Criterion D).

Associated Features Supporting Diagnosis

Although deficiencies in vitamins or minerals (e.g., zinc, iron) have been reported in some instances, often no specific biological abnormalities are found. In some cases, pica comes to clinical attention only following general medical complications (e.g., mechanical bowel problems; intestinal obstruction, such as that resulting from a bezoar; intestinal perforation; infections such as toxoplasmosis and toxocariasis as a result of ingesting feces or dirt; poisoning, such as by ingestion of lead-based paint).

Prevalence

The prevalence of pica is unclear. Among individuals with intellectual disability, the prevalence of pica appears to increase with the severity of the condition.

Development and Course

Onset of pica can occur in childhood, adolescence, or adulthood, although childhood onset is most commonly reported. Pica can occur in otherwise normally developing children, whereas in adults, it appears more likely to occur in the context of intellectual disability or other mental disorders. The eating of nonnutritive, nonfood substances may also manifest in pregnancy, when specific cravings (e.g., chalk or ice) might occur. The diagnosis of pica during pregnancy is only appropriate if such cravings lead to the ingestion of nonnutritive, nonfood substances to the extent that the eating of these substances poses potential medical risks. The course of the disorder can be protracted and can result in medical emergencies (e.g., intestinal obstruction, acute weight loss, poisoning). The disorder can potentially be fatal depending on substances ingested.

Risk and Prognostic Factors

Environmental.   Neglect, lack of supervision, and developmental delay can increase the risk for this condition.

Culture-Related Diagnostic Issues

In some populations, the eating of earth or other seemingly nonnutritive substances is believed to be of spiritual, medicinal, or other social value, or may be a culturally supported or socially normative practice. Such behavior does not warrant a diagnosis of pica (Criterion C).

Gender-Related Diagnostic Issues

Pica occurs in both males and females. It can occur in females during pregnancy; however, little is known about the course of pica in the postpartum period.

Diagnostic Markers

Abdominal flat plate radiography, ultrasound, and other scanning methods may reveal obstructions related to pica. Blood tests and other laboratory tests can be used to ascertain levels of poisoning or the nature of infection.

Functional Consequences of Pica

Pica can significantly impair physical functioning, but it is rarely the sole cause of impairment in social functioning. Pica often occurs with other disorders associated with impaired social functioning.

Differential Diagnosis

Eating of nonnutritive, nonfood substances may occur during the course of other mental disorders (e.g., autism spectrum disorder, schizophrenia) and in Kleine-Levin syndrome. In any such instance, an additional diagnosis of pica should be given only if the eating behavior is sufficiently persistent and severe to warrant additional clinical attention.

Anorexia nervosa.   Pica can usually be distinguished from the other feeding and eating disorders by the consumption of nonnutritive, nonfood substances. It is important to note, however, that some presentations of anorexia nervosa include ingestion of nonnutritive, nonfood substances, such as paper tissues, as a means of attempting to control appetite. In such cases, when the eating of nonnutritive, nonfood substances is primarily used as a means of weight control, anorexia nervosa should be the primary diagnosis.

Factitious disorder. Some individuals with factitious disorder may intentionally ingest foreign objects as part of the pattern of falsification of physical symptoms. In such instances, there is an element of deception that is consistent with deliberate induction of injury or disease.

Nonsuicidal self-injury and nonsuicidal self-injury behaviors in personality disorders. Some individuals may swallow potentially harmful items (e.g., pins, needles, knives) in the context of maladaptive behavior patterns associated with personality disorders or nonsuicidal self-injury.

Comorbidity

Disorders most commonly comorbid with pica are autism spectrum disorder and intellectual disability (intellectual developmental disorder), and, to a lesser degree, schizophrenia and obsessive-compulsive disorder. Pica can be associated with trichotillomania (hair-pulling disorder) and excoriation (skin-picking) disorder. In comorbid presentations, the hair or skin is typically ingested. Pica can also be associated with avoidant/restrictive food intake disorder, particularly in individuals with a strong sensory component to their presentation. When an individual is known to have pica, assessment should include consideration of the possibility of gastrointestinal complications, poisoning, infection, and nutritional deficiency.

Rumination Disorder

Diagnostic Criteria **307.53** (F98.21)

A. Repeated regurgitation of food over a period of at least 1 month. Regurgitated food may be re-chewed, re-swallowed, or spit out.
B. The repeated regurgitation is not attributable to an associated gastrointestinal or other medical condition (e.g., gastroesophageal reflux, pyloric stenosis).
C. The eating disturbance does not occur exclusively during the course of anorexia nervosa, bulimia nervosa, binge-eating disorder, or avoidant/restrictive food intake disorder.
D. If the symptoms occur in the context of another mental disorder (e.g., intellectual disability [intellectual developmental disorder] or another neurodevelopmental disorder), they are sufficiently severe to warrant additional clinical attention.

Specify if:
    In remission: After full criteria for rumination disorder were previously met, the criteria have not been met for a sustained period of time.

Diagnostic Features

The essential feature of rumination disorder is the repeated regurgitation of food occurring after feeding or eating over a period of at least 1 month (Criterion A). Previously swallowed food that may be partially digested is brought up into the mouth without apparent nausea, involuntary retching, or disgust. The food may be re-chewed and then ejected from the mouth or re-swallowed. Regurgitation in rumination disorder should be frequent, occurring at least several times per week, typically daily. The behavior is not better explained by an associated gastrointestinal or other medical condition (e.g., gastroesophageal reflux, pyloric stenosis) (Criterion B) and does not occur exclusively during the course of anorexia nervosa, bulimia nervosa, binge-eating disorder, or avoidant/restrictive food intake disorder (Criterion C). If the symptoms occur in the context of another mental disorder (e.g., intellectual disability [intellectual developmental disorder], neurodevelopmental disorder), they must be sufficiently severe to warrant additional clinical attention (Criterion D) and should represent a primary aspect of the individual's presentation requiring intervention. The disorder may be diagnosed across the life span, particularly in individuals who also have intellectual disability. Many individuals with rumination disorder can be directly observed engaging in the behavior by the clinician. In other instances diagnosis can be made on the basis of self-report or corroborative information from parents or caregivers. Individuals may describe the behavior as habitual or outside of their control.

Associated Features Supporting Diagnosis

Infants with rumination disorder display a characteristic position of straining and arching the back with the head held back, making sucking movements with their tongue. They may give the impression of gaining satisfaction from the activity. They may be irritable and hungry between episodes of regurgitation. Weight loss and failure to make expected weight gains are common features in infants with rumination disorder. Malnutrition may occur despite the infant's apparent hunger and the ingestion of relatively large amounts of food, particularly in severe cases, when regurgitation immediately follows each feeding episode and regurgitated food is expelled. Malnutrition might also occur in older children and adults, particularly when the regurgitation is accompanied by restriction of intake. Adolescents and adults may attempt to disguise the regurgitation behavior by placing a hand over the mouth or coughing. Some will avoid eating with others because of the acknowledged social undesirability of the behavior. This may extend to an avoidance of eating prior to social situations, such as work or school (e.g., avoiding breakfast because it may be followed by regurgitation).

Prevalence

Prevalence data for rumination disorder are inconclusive, but the disorder is commonly reported to be higher in certain groups, such as individuals with intellectual disability.

Development and Course

Onset of rumination disorder can occur in infancy, childhood, adolescence, or adulthood. The age at onset in infants is usually between ages 3 and 12 months. In infants, the disorder frequently remits spontaneously, but its course can be protracted and can result in medical emergencies (e.g., severe malnutrition). It can potentially be fatal, particularly in infancy. Rumination disorder can have an episodic course or occur continuously until treated. In infants, as well as in older individuals with intellectual disability (intellectual developmental disorder) or other neurodevelopmental disorders, the regurgitation and rumination behavior appears to have a self-soothing or self-stimulating function, similar to that of other repetitive motor behaviors such as head banging.

Risk and Prognostic Factors

Environmental. Psychosocial problems such as lack of stimulation, neglect, stressful life situations, and problems in the parent-child relationship may be predisposing factors in infants and young children.

Functional Consequences of Rumination Disorder

Malnutrition secondary to repeated regurgitation may be associated with growth delay and have a negative effect on development and learning potential. Some older individuals with rumination disorder deliberately restrict their food intake because of the social undesirability of regurgitation. They may therefore present with weight loss or low weight. In older children, adolescents, and adults, social functioning is more likely to be adversely affected.

Differential Diagnosis

Gastrointestinal conditions. It is important to differentiate regurgitation in rumination disorder from other conditions characterized by gastroesophageal reflux or vomiting. Conditions such as gastroparesis, pyloric stenosis, hiatal hernia, and Sandifer syndrome in infants should be ruled out by appropriate physical examinations and laboratory tests.

Anorexia nervosa and bulimia nervosa. Individuals with anorexia nervosa and bulimia nervosa may also engage in regurgitation with subsequent spitting out of food as a means of disposing of ingested calories because of concerns about weight gain.

Comorbidity

Regurgitation with associated rumination can occur in the context of a concurrent medical condition or another mental disorder (e.g., generalized anxiety disorder). When the regurgitation occurs in this context, a diagnosis of rumination disorder is appropriate only when the severity of the disturbance exceeds that routinely associated with such conditions or disorders and warrants additional clinical attention.

Avoidant/Restrictive Food Intake Disorder

Diagnostic Criteria **307.59** (F50.8)

A. An eating or feeding disturbance (e.g., apparent lack of interest in eating or food; avoidance based on the sensory characteristics of food; concern about aversive consequences of eating) as manifested by persistent failure to meet appropriate nutritional and/or energy needs associated with one (or more) of the following:

1. Significant weight loss (or failure to achieve expected weight gain or faltering growth in children).
2. Significant nutritional deficiency.
3. Dependence on enteral feeding or oral nutritional supplements.
4. Marked interference with psychosocial functioning.

B. The disturbance is not better explained by lack of available food or by an associated culturally sanctioned practice.
C. The eating disturbance does not occur exclusively during the course of anorexia nervosa or bulimia nervosa, and there is no evidence of a disturbance in the way in which one's body weight or shape is experienced.
D. The eating disturbance is not attributable to a concurrent medical condition or not better explained by another mental disorder. When the eating disturbance occurs in the context of another condition or disorder, the severity of the eating disturbance exceeds that routinely associated with the condition or disorder and warrants additional clinical attention.

Specify if:

In remission: After full criteria for avoidant/restrictive food intake disorder were previously met, the criteria have not been met for a sustained period of time.

Diagnostic Features

Avoidant/restrictive food intake disorder replaces and extends the DSM-IV diagnosis of feeding disorder of infancy or early childhood. The main diagnostic feature of avoidant/restrictive food intake disorder is avoidance or restriction of food intake (Criterion A) manifested by clinically significant failure to meet requirements for nutrition or insufficient energy intake through oral intake of food. One or more of the following key features must be present: significant weight loss, significant nutritional deficiency (or related health impact), dependence on enteral feeding or oral nutritional supplements, or marked interference with psychosocial functioning. The determination of whether weight loss is significant (Criterion A1) is a clinical judgment; instead of losing weight, children and adolescents who have not completed growth may not maintain weight or height increases along their developmental trajectory.

Determination of significant nutritional deficiency (Criterion A2) is also based on clinical assessment (e.g., assessment of dietary intake, physical examination, and laboratory testing), and related impact on physical health can be of a similar severity to that seen in anorexia nervosa (e.g., hypothermia, bradycardia, anemia). In severe cases, particularly in infants, malnutrition can be life threatening. "Dependence" on enteral feeding or oral nutritional supplements (Criterion A3) means that supplementary feeding is required to sustain adequate intake. Examples of individuals requiring supplementary feeding include infants with failure to thrive who require nasogastric tube feeding, children with neurodevelopmental disorders who are dependent on nutritionally complete supplements, and individuals who rely on gastrostomy tube feeding or complete oral nutrition supplements in the absence of an underlying medical condition. Inability to participate in normal social activities, such as eating with others, or to sustain relationships as a result of the disturbance would indicate marked interference with psychosocial functioning (Criterion A4).

Avoidant/restrictive food intake disorder does not include avoidance or restriction of food intake related to lack of availability of food or to cultural practices (e.g., religious fasting or normal dieting) (Criterion B), nor does it include developmentally normal behaviors (e.g., picky eating in toddlers, reduced intake in older adults). The disturbance is not better explained by excessive concern about body weight or shape (Criterion C) or by concurrent medical factors or mental disorders (Criterion D).

In some individuals, food avoidance or restriction may be based on the sensory characteristics of qualities of food, such as extreme sensitivity to appearance, color, smell, texture, temperature, or taste. Such behavior has been described as "restrictive eating," "selective eating," "choosy eating," "perseverant eating," "chronic food refusal," and "food neophobia" and may manifest as refusal to eat particular brands of foods or to tolerate the smell of food being eaten by others. Individuals with heightened sensory sensitivities associated with autism may show similar behaviors.

Food avoidance or restriction may also represent a conditioned negative response associated with food intake following, or in anticipation of, an aversive experience, such as choking; a traumatic investigation, usually involving the gastrointestinal tract (e.g., esophagoscopy); or repeated vomiting. The terms *functional dysphagia* and *globus hystericus* have also been used for such conditions.

Associated Features Supporting Diagnosis

Several features may be associated with food avoidance or reduced food intake, including a lack of interest in eating or food, leading to weight loss or faltering growth. Very young infants may present as being too sleepy, distressed, or agitated to feed. Infants and young children may not engage with the primary caregiver during feeding or communicate hunger in favor of other activities. In older children and adolescents, food avoidance or restriction may be associated with more generalized emotional difficulties that do not meet diagnostic criteria for an anxiety, depressive, or bipolar disorder, sometimes called "food avoidance emotional disorder."

Development and Course

Food avoidance or restriction associated with insufficient intake or lack of interest in eating most commonly develops in infancy or early childhood and may persist in adulthood. Likewise, avoidance based on sensory characteristics of food tends to arise in the first decade of life but may persist into adulthood. Avoidance related to aversive consequences can arise at any age. The scant literature regarding long-term outcomes suggests that food avoidance or restriction based on sensory aspects is relatively stable and long-standing, but when persisting into adulthood, such avoidance/restriction can be associated with relatively normal functioning. There is currently insufficient evidence directly linking avoidant/restrictive food intake disorder and subsequent onset of an eating disorder.

Infants with avoidant/restrictive food intake disorder may be irritable and difficult to console during feeding, or may appear apathetic and withdrawn. In some instances, parent-child interaction may contribute to the infant's feeding problem (e.g., presenting food inappropriately, or interpreting the infant's behavior as an act of aggression or rejection). Inadequate nutritional intake may exacerbate the associated features (e.g., irritability, developmental lags) and further contribute to feeding difficulties. Associated factors include infant temperament or developmental impairments that reduce an infant's responsiveness to feeding. Coexisting parental psychopathology, or child abuse or neglect, is suggested if feeding and weight improve in response to changing caregivers. In infants, children, and prepubertal adolescents, avoidant/restrictive food intake disorder may be associated with growth delay, and the resulting malnutrition negatively affects development and learning potential. In older children, adolescents, and adults, social functioning tends to be adversely affected. Regardless of the age, family function may be affected, with heightened stress at mealtimes and in other feeding or eating contexts involving friends and relatives.

Avoidant/restrictive food intake disorder manifests more commonly in children than in adults, and there may be a long delay between onset and clinical presentation. Triggers for presentation vary considerably and include physical, social, and emotional difficulties.

Risk and Prognostic Factors

Temperamental. Anxiety disorders, autism spectrum disorder, obsessive-compulsive disorder (OCD), and attention-deficit/hyperactivity disorder may increase risk for avoidant or restrictive feeding or eating behavior characteristic of the disorder.

Environmental. Environmental risk factors for avoidant/restrictive food intake disorder include familial anxiety. Higher rates of feeding disturbances may occur in children of mothers with eating disorders.

Genetic and physiological. History of gastrointestinal conditions, gastroesophageal reflux disease, vomiting, and a range of other medical problems has been associated with feeding and eating behaviors characteristic of avoidant/restrictive food intake disorder.

Culture-Related Diagnostic Issues

Presentations similar to avoidant/restrictive food intake disorder occur in various populations, including in the United States, Canada, Australia, and Europe. Avoidant/restrictive food intake disorder should not be diagnosed when avoidance of food intake is solely related to specific religious or cultural practices.

Gender-Related Diagnostic Issues

Avoidant/restrictive food intake disorder is equally common in males and females in infancy and early childhood, but avoidant/restrictive food intake disorder comorbid with autism spectrum disorder has a male predominance. Food avoidance or restriction related to altered sensory sensitivities can occur in some physiological conditions, most notably pregnancy, but is not usually extreme and does not meet full criteria for the disorder.

Diagnostic Markers

Diagnostic markers include malnutrition, low weight, growth delay, and the need for artificial nutrition in the absence of any clear medical condition other than poor intake.

Functional Consequences of Avoidant/Restrictive Food Intake Disorder

Associated developmental and functional limitations include impairment of physical development and social difficulties that can have a significant negative impact on family function.

Differential Diagnosis

Appetite loss preceding restricted intake is a nonspecific symptom that can accompany a number of mental diagnoses. Avoidant/restrictive food intake disorder can be diagnosed concurrently with the disorders below if all criteria are met, and the eating disturbance requires specific clinical attention.

Other medical conditions (e.g., gastrointestinal disease, food allergies and intolerances, occult malignancies).   Restriction of food intake may occur in other medical conditions, especially those with ongoing symptoms such as vomiting, loss of appetite, nausea, abdominal pain, or diarrhea. A diagnosis of avoidant/restrictive food intake disorder requires that the disturbance of intake is beyond that directly accounted for by physical symptoms consistent with a medical condition; the eating disturbance may also persist after being triggered by a medical condition and following resolution of the medical condition.

Underlying medical or comorbid mental conditions may complicate feeding and eating. Because older individuals, postsurgical patients, and individuals receiving chemotherapy often lose their appetite, an additional diagnosis of avoidant/restrictive food intake disorder requires that the eating disturbance is a primary focus for intervention.

Specific neurological/neuromuscular, structural, or congenital disorders and conditions associated with feeding difficulties.   Feeding difficulties are common in a number of congenital and neurological conditions often related to problems with oral/esophageal/pharyngeal structure and function, such as hypotonia of musculature, tongue protrusion, and unsafe swallowing. Avoidant/restrictive food intake disorder can be diagnosed in individuals with such presentations as long as all diagnostic criteria are met.

Reactive attachment disorder.   Some degree of withdrawal is characteristic of reactive attachment disorder and can lead to a disturbance in the caregiver-child relationship that can affect feeding and the child's intake. Avoidant/restrictive food intake disorder should be diagnosed concurrently only if all criteria are met for both disorders and the feeding disturbance is a primary focus for intervention.

Autism spectrum disorder.   Individuals with autism spectrum disorder often present with rigid eating behaviors and heightened sensory sensitivities. However, these features do not always result in the level of impairment that would be required for a diagnosis of avoidant/restrictive food intake disorder. Avoidant/restrictive food intake disorder should be diagnosed concurrently only if all criteria are met for both disorders and when the eating disturbance requires specific treatment.

Specific phobia, social anxiety disorder (social phobia), and other anxiety disorders. Specific phobia, other type, specifies "situations that may lead to choking or vomiting" and can represent the primary trigger for the fear, anxiety, or avoidance required for diagnosis. Distinguishing specific phobia from avoidant/restrictive food intake disorder can be difficult when a fear of choking or vomiting has resulted in food avoidance. Although avoidance or restriction of food intake secondary to a pronounced fear of choking or vomiting can be conceptualized as specific phobia, in situations when the eating problem becomes the primary focus of clinical attention, avoidant/restrictive food intake disorder becomes the appropriate diagnosis. In social anxiety disorder, the individual may present with a fear of being observed by others while eating, which can also occur in avoidant/restrictive food intake disorder.

Anorexia nervosa. Restriction of energy intake relative to requirements leading to significantly low body weight is a core feature of anorexia nervosa. However, individuals with anorexia nervosa also display a fear of gaining weight or of becoming fat, or persistent behavior that interferes with weight gain, as well as specific disturbances in relation to perception and experience of their own body weight and shape. These features are not present in avoidant/restrictive food intake disorder, and the two disorders should not be diagnosed concurrently. Differential diagnosis between avoidant/restrictive food intake disorder and anorexia nervosa may be difficult, especially in late childhood and early adolescence, because these disorders may share a number of common symptoms (e.g., food avoidance, low weight). Differential diagnosis is also potentially difficult in individuals with anorexia nervosa who deny any fear of fatness but nonetheless engage in persistent behaviors that prevent weight gain and who do not recognize the medical seriousness of their low weight—a presentation sometimes termed "non-fat phobic anorexia nervosa". Full consideration of symptoms, course, and family history is advised, and diagnosis may be best made in the context of a clinical relationship over time. In some individuals, avoidant/restrictive food intake disorder might precede the onset of anorexia nervosa.

Obsessive-compulsive disorder. Individuals with obsessive-compulsive disorder may present with avoidance or restriction of intake in relation to preoccupations with food or ritualized eating behavior. Avoidant/restrictive food intake disorder should be diagnosed concurrently only if all criteria are met for both disorders and when the aberrant eating is a major aspect of the clinical presentation requiring specific intervention.

Major depressive disorder. In major depressive disorder, appetite might be affected to such an extent that individuals present with significantly restricted food intake, usually in relation to overall energy intake and often associated with weight loss. Usually appetite loss and related reduction of intake abate with resolution of mood problems. Avoidant/restrictive food intake disorder should only be used concurrently if full criteria are met for both disorders and when the eating disturbance requires specific treatment.

Schizophrenia spectrum disorders. Individuals with schizophrenia, delusional disorder, or other psychotic disorders may exhibit odd eating behaviors, avoidance of specific foods because of delusional beliefs, or other manifestations of avoidant or re-strictive intake. In some cases, delusional beliefs may contribute to a concern about negative consequences of ingesting certain foods. Avoidant/restrictive food intake disorder should be used concurrently only if all criteria are met for both disorders and when the eating disturbance requires specific treatment.

Factitious disorder or factitious disorder imposed on another.   Avoidant/restrictive food intake disorder should be differentiated from factitious disorder or factitious disorder imposed on another. In order to assume the sick role, some individuals with factitious disorder may intentionally describe diets that are much more restrictive than those they are actually able to consume, as well as complications of such behavior, such as a need for enteral feedings or nutritional supplements, an inability to tolerate a normal range of foods, and/or an inability to participate normally in age-appropriate situations involving food. The presentation may be impressively dramatic and engag-ing, and the symptoms reported inconsistently. In factitious disorder imposed on an-other, the caregiver describes symptoms consistent with avoidant/restrictive food intake disorder and may induce physical symptoms such as failure to gain weight. As with any diagnosis of factitious disorder imposed on another, the caregiver receives the diagnosis rather than the affected individual, and diagnosis should be made only on the basis of a careful, comprehensive assessment of the affected individual, the care-giver, and their interaction.

Comorbidity

The most commonly observed disorders comorbid with avoidant/restrictive food in-take disorder are anxiety disorders, obsessive-compulsive disorder, and neurodevelop-mental disorders (specifically autism spectrum disorder, attention-deficit/hyperactivity disorder, and intellectual disability [intellectual developmental disorder]).

Anorexia Nervosa

Diagnostic Criteria

A. Restriction of energy intake relative to requirements, leading to a significantly low body weight in the context of age, sex, developmental trajectory, and physical health. *Significantly low weight* is defined as a weight that is less than minimally normal or, for children and adolescents, less than that minimally expected.

B. Intense fear of gaining weight or of becoming fat, or persistent behavior that inter-feres with weight gain, even though at a significantly low weight.

C. Disturbance in the way in which one's body weight or shape is experienced, undue influence of body weight or shape on self-evaluation, or persistent lack of recogni-tion of the seriousness of the current low body weight.

Coding note: The ICD-9-CM code for anorexia nervosa is **307.1,** which is assigned regardless of the subtype. The ICD-10-CM code depends on the subtype (see below).

Specify whether:

(F50.01) Restricting type: During the last 3 months, the individual has not en-gaged in recurrent episodes of binge eating or purging behavior (i.e., self-induced vomiting or the misuse of laxatives, diuretics, or enemas). This subtype describes presentations in which weight loss is accomplished primarily through dieting, fasting, and/or excessive exercise.

(F50.02) Binge-eating/purging type: During the last 3 months, the individual has engaged in recurrent episodes of binge eating or purging behavior (i.e., self-induced vomiting or the misuse of laxatives, diuretics, or enemas).

Specify if:

In partial remission: After full criteria for anorexia nervosa were previously met, Criterion A (low body weight) has not been met for a sustained period, but either Criterion B (intense fear of gaining weight or becoming fat or behavior that interferes with weight gain) or Criterion C (disturbances in self-perception of weight and shape) is still met.

In full remission: After full criteria for anorexia nervosa were previously met, none of the criteria have been met for a sustained period of time.

Specify current severity:

The minimum level of severity is based, for adults, on current body mass index (BMI) (see below) or, for children and adolescents, on BMI percentile. The ranges below are derived from World Health Organization categories for thinness in adults; for children and adolescents, corresponding BMI percentiles should be used. The level of severity may be increased to reflect clinical symptoms, the degree of functional disability, and the need for supervision.

Mild: BMI ≥ 17 kg/m^2
Moderate: BMI 16–16.99 kg/m^2
Severe: BMI 15–15.99 kg/m^2
Extreme: BMI < 15 kg/m^2

Subtypes

Most individuals with the binge-eating/purging type of anorexia nervosa who binge eat also purge through self-induced vomiting or the misuse of laxatives, diuretics, or enemas. Some individuals with this subtype of anorexia nervosa do not binge eat but do regularly purge after the consumption of small amounts of food.

Crossover between the subtypes over the course of the disorder is not uncommon; therefore, subtype description should be used to describe current symptoms rather than longitudinal course.

Diagnostic Features

There are three essential features of anorexia nervosa: persistent energy intake restriction; intense fear of gaining weight or of becoming fat, or persistent behavior that interferes with weight gain; and a disturbance in self-perceived weight or shape. The individual maintains a body weight that is below a minimally normal level for age, sex, developmental trajectory, and physical health (Criterion A). Individuals' body weights frequently meet this criterion following a significant weight loss, but among children and adolescents, there may alternatively be failure to make expected weight gain or to maintain a normal developmental trajectory (i.e., while growing in height) instead of weight loss.

Criterion A requires that the individual's weight be significantly low (i.e., less than minimally normal or, for children and adolescents, less than that minimally expected). Weight assessment can be challenging because normal weight range differs among individuals, and different thresholds have been published defining thinness or underweight status. Body mass index (BMI; calculated as weight in kilograms/height in meters^2) is a useful measure to assess body weight for height. For adults, a BMI of 18.5 kg/m^2 has been employed by the Centers for Disease Control and Prevention (CDC) and the World Health Organization (WHO) as the lower limit of normal body weight. Therefore, most adults with a BMI greater than or equal to 18.5 kg/m^2 would not be considered to have a significantly low body weight. On the other hand, a BMI of lower than 17.0 kg/m^2 has been considered by the WHO to indicate moderate or severe thinness; therefore, an individual with a BMI less than 17.0 kg/m^2 would likely be considered to have a significantly low weight. An adult with a BMI between 17.0 and 18.5 kg/m^2, or even above 18.5 kg/m^2, might be considered to have a significantly low weight if clinical history or other physiological information supports this judgment.

For children and adolescents, determining a BMI-for-age percentile is useful (see, e.g., the CDC BMI percentile calculator for children and teenagers, . As for adults, it is not possible to provide definitive standards for judging whether a child's or an adolescent's weight is significantly low, and variations in developmental trajectories among youth limit the utility of simple numerical guidelines. The CDC has used a BMI-for-age below the 5th percentile as suggesting underweight; however, children and adolescents with a BMI above this benchmark may be judged to be significantly underweight in light of failure to maintain their expected growth trajectory. In summary, in determining whether Criterion A is met, the clinician should consider available numerical guidelines, as well as the individual's body build, weight history, and any physiological disturbances.

Individuals with this disorder typically display an intense fear of gaining weight or of becoming fat (Criterion B). This intense fear of becoming fat is usually not alleviated by weight loss. In fact, concern about weight gain may increase even as weight falls. Younger individuals with anorexia nervosa, as well as some adults, may not recognize or acknowledge a fear of weight gain. In the absence of another explanation for the significantly low weight, clinician inference drawn from collateral history, observational data, physical and laboratory findings, or longitudinal course either indicating a fear of weight gain or supporting persistent behaviors that prevent it may be used to establish Criterion B.

The experience and significance of body weight and shape are distorted in these individuals (Criterion C). Some individuals feel globally overweight. Others realize that they are thin but are still concerned that certain body parts, particularly the abdomen, buttocks, and thighs, are "too fat." They may employ a variety of techniques to evaluate their body size or weight, including frequent weighing, obsessive measuring of body parts, and persistent use of a mirror to check for perceived areas of "fat." The self-esteem of individuals with anorexia nervosa is highly dependent on their perceptions of body shape and weight. Weight loss is often viewed as an impressive achievement and a sign of extraordinary self-discipline, whereas weight gain is perceived as an unacceptable failure of self-control. Although some individuals with this disorder may acknowledge being thin, they often do not recognize the serious medical implications of their malnourished state.

Often, the individual is brought to professional attention by family members after marked weight loss (or failure to make expected weight gains) has occurred. If individuals seek help on their own, it is usually because of distress over the somatic and psychological sequelae of starvation. It is rare for an individual with anorexia nervosa to complain of weight loss per se. In fact, individuals with anorexia nervosa frequently either lack insight into or deny the problem. It is therefore often important to obtain information from family members or other sources to evaluate the history of weight loss and other features of the illness.

Associated Features Supporting Diagnosis

The semi-starvation of anorexia nervosa, and the purging behaviors sometimes associated with it, can result in significant and potentially life-threatening medical conditions. The nutritional compromise associated with this disorder affects most major organ systems and can produce a variety of disturbances. Physiological disturbances, including amenorrhea and vital sign abnormalities, are common. While most of the physiological disturbances associated with malnutrition are reversible with nutritional rehabilitation, some, including loss of bone mineral density, are often not completely reversible. Behaviors such as self-induced vomiting and misuse of laxatives, diuretics, and enemas may cause a number of disturbances that lead to abnormal laboratory findings; however, some individuals with anorexia nervosa exhibit no laboratory abnormalities.

When seriously underweight, many individuals with anorexia nervosa have depressive signs and symptoms such as depressed mood, social withdrawal, irritability, insomnia, and diminished interest in sex. Because these features are also observed in individuals without anorexia nervosa who are significantly undernourished, many of the depressive features may be secondary to the physiological sequelae of semi-starvation, although they may also be sufficiently severe to warrant an additional diagnosis of major depressive disorder.

Obsessive-compulsive features, both related and unrelated to food, are often prominent. Most individuals with anorexia nervosa are preoccupied with thoughts of food. Some collect recipes or hoard food. Observations of behaviors associated with other forms of starvation suggest that obsessions and compulsions related to food may be exacerbated by undernutrition. When individuals with anorexia nervosa exhibit obsessions and compulsions that are not related to food, body shape, or weight, an additional diagnosis of OCD may be warranted.

Other features sometimes associated with anorexia nervosa include concerns about eating in public, feelings of ineffectiveness, a strong desire to control one's environment, inflexible thinking, limited social spontaneity, and overly restrained emotional expression. Compared with individuals with anorexia nervosa, restricting type, those with binge-eating/purging type have higher rates of impulsivity and are more likely to abuse alcohol and other drugs.

A subgroup of individuals with anorexia nervosa show excessive levels of physical activity. Increases in physical activity often precede onset of the disorder, and over the course of the disorder increased activity accelerates weight loss. During treatment, excessive activity may be difficult to control, thereby jeopardizing weight recovery.

Individuals with anorexia nervosa may misuse medications, such as by manipulating dosage, in order to achieve weight loss or avoid weight gain. Individuals with diabetes mellitus may omit or reduce insulin doses in order to minimize carbohydrate metabolism.

Prevalence

The 12-month prevalence of anorexia nervosa among young females is approximately 0.4%. Less is known about prevalence among males, but anorexia nervosa is far less common in males than in females, with clinical populations generally reflecting approximately a 10:1 female-to-male ratio.

Development and Course

Anorexia nervosa commonly begins during adolescence or young adulthood. It rarely begins before puberty or after age 40, but cases of both early and late onset have been described. The onset of this disorder is often associated with a stressful life event, such as leaving home for college. The course and outcome of anorexia nervosa are highly variable. Younger individuals may manifest atypical features, including denying "fear of fat." Older individuals more likely have a longer duration of illness, and their clinical presentation may include more signs and symptoms of long-standing disorder. Clinicians should not exclude anorexia nervosa from the differential diagnosis solely on the basis of older age.

Many individuals have a period of changed eating behavior prior to full criteria for the disorder being met. Some individuals with anorexia nervosa recover fully after a single episode, with some exhibiting a fluctuating pattern of weight gain followed by relapse, and others experiencing a chronic course over many years. Hospitalization may be required to restore weight and to address medical complications. Most individuals with anorexia nervosa experience remission within 5 years of presentation. Among individuals admitted to hospitals, overall remission rates may be lower. The crude mortality rate (CMR) for anorexia nervosa is approximately 5% per decade. Death most commonly results from medical complications associated with the disorder itself or from suicide.

Risk and Prognostic Factors

Temperamental.   Individuals who develop anxiety disorders or display obsessional traits in childhood are at increased risk of developing anorexia nervosa.

Environmental.   Historical and cross-cultural variability in the prevalence of anorexia nervosa supports its association with cultures and settings in which thinness is valued. Occupations and avocations that encourage thinness, such as modeling and elite athletics, are also associated with increased risk.

Genetic and physiological.   There is an increased risk of anorexia nervosa and bulimia nervosa among first-degree biological relatives of individuals with the disorder. An increased risk of bipolar and depressive disorders has also been found among first-degree relatives of individuals with anorexia nervosa, particularly relatives of individuals with the binge-eating/purging type. Concordance rates for anorexia nervosa in monozygotic twins are significantly higher than those for dizygotic twins. A range of brain abnormalities has been described in anorexia nervosa using functional imaging technologies (functional magnetic resonance imaging, positron emission tomography). The degree to which these findings reflect changes associated with malnutrition versus primary abnormalities associated with the disorder is unclear.

Culture-Related Diagnostic Issues

Anorexia nervosa occurs across culturally and socially diverse populations, although available evidence suggests cross-cultural variation in its occurrence and presentation. Anorexia nervosa is probably most prevalent in post-industrialized, high-income countries such as in the United States, many European countries, Australia, New Zealand, and Japan, but its incidence in most low- and middle-income countries is uncertain. Whereas the prevalence of anorexia nervosa appears comparatively low among Latinos, African Americans, and Asians in the United States, clinicians should be aware that mental health service utilization among individuals with an eating disorder is significantly lower in these ethnic groups and that the low rates may reflect an ascertainment bias. The presentation of weight concerns among individuals with eating and feeding disorders varies substantially across cultural contexts. The absence of an expressed intense fear of weight gain, sometimes referred to as "fat phobia," appears to be relatively more common in populations in Asia, where the rationale for dietary restriction is commonly related to a more culturally sanctioned complaint such as gastrointestinal discomfort. Within the United States, presentations without a stated intense fear of weight gain may be comparatively more common among Latino groups.

Diagnostic Markers

The following laboratory abnormalities may be observed in anorexia nervosa; their presence may serve to increase diagnostic confidence.

Hematology. Leukopenia is common, with the loss of all cell types but usually with apparent lymphocytosis. Mild anemia can occur, as well as thrombocytopenia and, rarely, bleeding problems.

Serum chemistry. Dehydration may be reflected by an elevated blood urea nitrogen level. Hypercholesterolemia is common. Hepatic enzyme levels may be elevated. Hypomagnesemia, hypozincemia, hypophosphatemia, and hyperamylasemia are occasionally observed. Self-induced vomiting may lead to metabolic alkalosis (elevated serum bicarbonate), hypochloremia, and hypokalemia; laxative abuse may cause a mild metabolic acidosis.

Endocrine. Serum thyroxine (T_4) levels are usually in the low-normal range; triiodothyronine (T_3) levels are decreased, while reverse T_3 levels are elevated. Females have low serum estrogen levels, whereas males have low levels of serum testosterone.

Electrocardiography. Sinus bradycardia is common, and, rarely, arrhythmias are noted. Significant prolongation of the QTc interval is observed in some individuals.

Bone mass.   Low bone mineral density, with specific areas of osteopenia or osteoporosis, is often seen. The risk of fracture is significantly elevated.

Electroencephalography.   Diffuse abnormalities, reflecting a metabolic encephalopathy, may result from significant fluid and electrolyte disturbances.

Resting energy expenditure.   There is often a significant reduction in resting energy expenditure.

Physical signs and symptoms.   Many of the physical signs and symptoms of anorexia nervosa are attributable to starvation. Amenorrhea is commonly present and appears to be an indicator of physiological dysfunction. If present, amenorrhea is usually a consequence of the weight loss, but in a minority of individuals it may actually precede the weight loss. In prepubertal females, menarche may be delayed. In addition to amenorrhea, there may be complaints of constipation, abdominal pain, cold intolerance, lethargy, and excess energy.

The most remarkable finding on physical examination is emaciation. Commonly, there is also significant hypotension, hypothermia, and bradycardia. Some individuals develop lanugo, a fine downy body hair. Some develop peripheral edema, especially during weight restoration or upon cessation of laxative and diuretic abuse. Rarely, petechiae or ecchymoses, usually on the extremities, may indicate a bleeding diathesis. Some individuals evidence a yellowing of the skin associated with hypercarotenemia. As may be seen in individuals with bulimia nervosa, individuals with anorexia nervosa who self-induce vomiting may have hypertrophy of the salivary glands, particularly the parotid glands, as well as dental enamel erosion. Some individuals may have scars or calluses on the dorsal surface of the hand from repeated contact with the teeth while inducing vomiting.

Suicide Risk

Suicide risk is elevated in anorexia nervosa, with rates reported as 12 per 100,000 per year. Comprehensive evaluation of individuals with anorexia nervosa should include assessment of suicide-related ideation and behaviors as well as other risk factors for suicide, including a history of suicide attempt(s).

Functional Consequences of Anorexia Nervosa

Individuals with anorexia nervosa may exhibit a range of functional limitations associated with the disorder. While some individuals remain active in social and professional functioning, others demonstrate significant social isolation and/or failure to fulfill academic or career potential.

Differential Diagnosis

Other possible causes of either significantly low body weight or significant weight loss should be considered in the differential diagnosis of anorexia nervosa, especially when the presenting features are atypical (e.g., onset after age 40 years).

Medical conditions (e.g., gastrointestinal disease, hyperthyroidism, occult malignancies, and acquired immunodeficiency syndrome [AIDS]).   Serious weight loss may occur in medical conditions, but individuals with these disorders usually do not also manifest a disturbance in the way their body weight or shape is experienced or an intense fear of weight gain or persist in behaviors that interfere with appropriate weight gain. Acute weight loss associated with a medical condition can occasionally be followed by the onset or recurrence of anorexia nervosa, which can initially be masked by the comorbid medical condition. Rarely, anorexia nervosa develops after bariatric surgery for obesity.

Major depressive disorder. In major depressive disorder, severe weight loss may occur, but most individuals with major depressive disorder do not have either a desire for excessive weight loss or an intense fear of gaining weight.

Schizophrenia. Individuals with schizophrenia may exhibit odd eating behavior and occasionally experience significant weight loss, but they rarely show the fear of gaining weight and the body image disturbance required for a diagnosis of anorexia nervosa.

Substance use disorders. Individuals with substance use disorders may experience low weight due to poor nutritional intake but generally do not fear gaining weight and do not manifest body image disturbance. Individuals who abuse substances that reduce appetite (e.g., cocaine, stimulants) and who also endorse fear of weight gain should be carefully evaluated for the possibility of comorbid anorexia nervosa, given that the substance use may represent a persistent behavior that interferes with weight gain (Criterion B).

Social anxiety disorder (social phobia), obsessive-compulsive disorder, and body dysmorphic disorder. Some of the features of anorexia nervosa overlap with the criteria for social phobia, OCD, and body dysmorphic disorder. Specifically, individuals may feel humiliated or embarrassed to be seen eating in public, as in social phobia; may exhibit obsessions and compulsions related to food, as in OCD; or may be preoccupied with an imagined defect in bodily appearance, as in body dysmorphic disorder. If the individual with anorexia nervosa has social fears that are limited to eating behavior alone, the diagnosis of social phobia should not be made, but social fears unrelated to eating behavior (e.g., excessive fear of speaking in public) may warrant an additional diagnosis of social phobia. Similarly, an additional diagnosis of OCD should be considered only if the individual exhibits obsessions and compulsions unrelated to food (e.g., an excessive fear of contamination), and an additional diagnosis of body dysmorphic disorder should be considered only if the distortion is unrelated to body shape and size (e.g., preoccupation that one's nose is too big).

Bulimia nervosa. Individuals with bulimia nervosa exhibit recurrent episodes of binge eating, engage in inappropriate behavior to avoid weight gain (e.g., self-induced vomiting), and are overly concerned with body shape and weight. However, unlike individuals with anorexia nervosa, binge-eating/purging type, individuals with bulimia nervosa maintain body weight at or above a minimally normal level.

Avoidant/restrictive food intake disorder. Individuals with this disorder may exhibit significant weight loss or significant nutritional deficiency, but they do not have a fear of gaining weight or of becoming fat, nor do they have a disturbance in the way they experience their body shape and weight.

Comorbidity

Bipolar, depressive, and anxiety disorders commonly co-occur with anorexia nervosa. Many individuals with anorexia nervosa report the presence of either an anxiety disorder or symptoms prior to onset of their eating disorder. OCD is described in some individuals with anorexia nervosa, especially those with the restricting type. Alcohol use disorder and other substance use disorders may also be comorbid with anorexia nervosa, especially among those with the binge-eating/purging type.

Bulimia Nervosa

Diagnostic Criteria   **307.51 (F50.2)**

A. Recurrent episodes of binge eating. An episode of binge eating is characterized by both of the following:

1. Eating, in a discrete period of time (e.g., within any 2-hour period), an amount of food that is definitely larger than what most individuals would eat in a similar period of time under similar circumstances.
2. A sense of lack of control over eating during the episode (e.g., a feeling that one cannot stop eating or control what or how much one is eating).

B. Recurrent inappropriate compensatory behaviors in order to prevent weight gain, such as self-induced vomiting; misuse of laxatives, diuretics, or other medications; fasting; or excessive exercise.

C. The binge eating and inappropriate compensatory behaviors both occur, on average, at least once a week for 3 months.

D. Self-evaluation is unduly influenced by body shape and weight.

E. The disturbance does not occur exclusively during episodes of anorexia nervosa.

Specify if:

In partial remission: After full criteria for bulimia nervosa were previously met, some, but not all, of the criteria have been met for a sustained period of time.

In full remission: After full criteria for bulimia nervosa were previously met, none of the criteria have been met for a sustained period of time.

Specify current severity:

The minimum level of severity is based on the frequency of inappropriate compensatory behaviors (see below). The level of severity may be increased to reflect other symptoms and the degree of functional disability.

Mild: An average of 1–3 episodes of inappropriate compensatory behaviors per week.

Moderate: An average of 4–7 episodes of inappropriate compensatory behaviors per week.

Severe: An average of 8–13 episodes of inappropriate compensatory behaviors per week.

Extreme: An average of 14 or more episodes of inappropriate compensatory behaviors per week.

Diagnostic Features

There are three essential features of bulimia nervosa: recurrent episodes of binge eating (Criterion A), recurrent inappropriate compensatory behaviors to prevent weight gain (Criterion B), and self-evaluation that is unduly influenced by body shape and weight (Criterion D). To qualify for the diagnosis, the binge eating and inappropriate compensatory behaviors must occur, on average, at least once per week for 3 months (Criterion C).

An "episode of binge eating" is defined as eating, in a discrete period of time, an amount of food that is definitely larger than most individuals would eat in a similar period of time under similar circumstances (Criterion A1). The context in which the eating occurs may affect the clinician's estimation of whether the intake is excessive. For example, a quantity of food that might be regarded as excessive for a typical meal might be considered normal during a celebration or holiday meal. A "discrete period of time" refers to a limited period, usually less than 2 hours. A single episode of binge eating need not be restricted to one setting. For example, an individual may begin a binge in a restaurant and then continue to eat on returning home. Continual snacking on small amounts of food throughout the day would not be considered an eating binge.

An occurrence of excessive food consumption must be accompanied by a sense of lack of control (Criterion A2) to be considered an episode of binge eating. An indicator of loss of control is the inability to refrain from eating or to stop eating once started. Some individuals describe a dissociative quality during, or following, the binge-eating episodes. The impairment in control associated with binge eating may not be absolute; for example, an individual may continue binge eating while the telephone is ringing but will cease if a roommate or spouse unexpectedly enters the room. Some individuals report that their binge-eating episodes are no longer characterized by an acute feeling of loss of control but rather by a more generalized pattern of uncontrolled eating. If individuals report that they have abandoned efforts to control their eating, loss of control should be considered as present. Binge eating can also be planned in some instances.

The type of food consumed during binges varies both across individuals and for a given individual. Binge eating appears to be characterized more by an abnormality in the amount of food consumed than by a craving for a specific nutrient. However, during binges, individuals tend to eat foods they would otherwise avoid.

Individuals with bulimia nervosa are typically ashamed of their eating problems and attempt to conceal their symptoms. Binge eating usually occurs in secrecy or as inconspicuously as possible. The binge eating often continues until the individual is uncomfortably, or even painfully, full. The most common antecedent of binge eating is negative affect. Other triggers include interpersonal stressors; dietary restraint; negative feelings related to body weight, body shape, and food; and boredom. Binge eating may minimize or mitigate factors that precipitated the episode in the short-term, but negative self-evaluation and dysphoria often are the delayed consequences.

Another essential feature of bulimia nervosa is the recurrent use of inappropriate compensatory behaviors to prevent weight gain, collectively referred to as *purge behaviors* or *purging* (Criterion B). Many individuals with bulimia nervosa employ several methods to compensate for binge eating. Vomiting is the most common inappropriate compensatory behavior. The immediate effects of vomiting include relief from physical discomfort and reduction of fear of gaining weight. In some cases, vomiting becomes a goal in itself, and the individual will binge eat in order to vomit or will vomit after eating a small amount of food. Individuals with bulimia nervosa may use a variety of methods to induce vomiting, including the use of fingers or instruments to stimulate the gag reflex. Individuals generally become adept at inducing vomiting and are eventually able to vomit at will. Rarely, individuals consume syrup of ipecac to induce vomiting. Other purging behaviors include the misuse of laxatives and diuretics. A number of other compensatory methods may also be used in rare cases. Individuals with bulimia nervosa may misuse enemas following episodes of binge eating, but this is seldom the sole compensatory method employed. Individuals with this disorder may take thyroid hormone in an attempt to avoid weight gain. Individuals with diabetes mellitus and bulimia nervosa may omit or reduce insulin doses in order to reduce the metabolism of food consumed during eating binges. Individuals with bulimia nervosa may fast for a day or more or exercise excessively in an attempt to prevent weight gain. Exercise may be considered excessive when it significantly interferes with important activities, when it occurs at inappropriate times or in inappropriate settings, or when the individual continues to exercise despite injury or other medical complications.

Individuals with bulimia nervosa place an excessive emphasis on body shape or weight in their self-evaluation, and these factors are typically extremely important in determining self-esteem (Criterion D). Individuals with this disorder may closely resemble those with anorexia nervosa in their fear of gaining weight, in their desire to lose weight, and in the level of dissatisfaction with their bodies. However, a diagnosis of bulimia nervosa should not be given when the disturbance occurs only during episodes of anorexia nervosa (Criterion E).

Associated Features Supporting Diagnosis

Individuals with bulimia nervosa typically are within the normal weight or overweight range (body mass index [BMI] ≥ 18.5 and < 30 in adults). The disorder occurs but is uncommon among obese individuals. Between eating binges, individuals with bulimia nervosa typically restrict their total caloric consumption and preferentially select low-calorie ("diet") foods while avoiding foods that they perceive to be fattening or likely to trigger a binge.

Menstrual irregularity or amenorrhea often occurs among females with bulimia nervosa; it is uncertain whether such disturbances are related to weight fluctuations, to nutritional deficiencies, or to emotional distress. The fluid and electrolyte disturbances resulting from the purging behavior are sometimes sufficiently severe to constitute medically serious problems. Rare but potentially fatal complications include esophageal tears, gastric rupture, and cardiac arrhythmias. Serious cardiac and skeletal myopathies have been reported among individuals following repeated use of syrup of ipecac to induce vomiting. Individuals who chronically abuse laxatives may become dependent on their use to stimulate bowel movements. Gastrointestinal symptoms are commonly associated with bulimia nervosa, and rectal prolapse has also been reported among individuals with this disorder.

Prevalence

Twelve-month prevalence of bulimia nervosa among young females is 1%–1.5%. Point prevalence is highest among young adults since the disorder peaks in older adolescence and young adulthood. Less is known about the point prevalence of bulimia nervosa in males, but bulimia nervosa is far less common in males than it is in females, with an approximately 10:1 female-to-male ratio.

Development and Course

Bulimia nervosa commonly begins in adolescence or young adulthood. Onset before puberty or after age 40 is uncommon. The binge eating frequently begins during or after an episode of dieting to lose weight. Experiencing multiple stressful life events also can precipitate onset of bulimia nervosa.

Disturbed eating behavior persists for at least several years in a high percentage of clinic samples. The course may be chronic or intermittent, with periods of remission alternating with recurrences of binge eating. However, over longer-term follow-up, the symptoms of many individuals appear to diminish with or without treatment, although treatment clearly impacts outcome. Periods of remission longer than 1 year are associated with better long-term outcome.

Significantly elevated risk for mortality (all-cause and suicide) has been reported for individuals with bulimia nervosa. The CMR (crude mortality rate) for bulimia nervosa is nearly 2% per decade.

Diagnostic cross-over from initial bulimia nervosa to anorexia nervosa occurs in a minority of cases (10%–15%). Individuals who do experience cross-over to anorexia nervosa commonly will revert back to bulimia nervosa or have multiple occurrences of cross-overs between these disorders. A subset of individuals with bulimia nervosa continue to binge eat but no longer engage in inappropriate compensatory behaviors, and therefore their symptoms meet criteria for binge-eating disorder or other specified eating disorder. Diagnosis should be based on the current (i.e., past 3 months) clinical presentation.

Risk and Prognostic Factors

Temperamental.   Weight concerns, low self-esteem, depressive symptoms, social anxiety disorder, and overanxious disorder of childhood are associated with increased risk for the development of bulimia nervosa.

Environmental.   Internalization of a thin body ideal has been found to increase risk for developing weight concerns, which in turn increase risk for the development of bulimia nervosa. Individuals who experienced childhood sexual or physical abuse are at increased risk for developing bulimia nervosa.

Genetic and physiological.   Childhood obesity and early pubertal maturation increase risk for bulimia nervosa. Familial transmission of bulimia nervosa may be present, as well as genetic vulnerabilities for the disorder.

Course modifiers.   Severity of psychiatric comorbidity predicts worse long-term outcome of bulimia nervosa.

Culture-Related Diagnostic Issues

Bulimia nervosa has been reported to occur with roughly similar frequencies in most industrialized countries, including the United States, Canada, many European countries, Australia, Japan, New Zealand, and South Africa. In clinical studies of bulimia nervosa in the United States, individuals presenting with this disorder are primarily white. However, the disorder also occurs in other ethnic groups and with prevalence comparable to estimated prevalences observed in white samples.

Gender-Related Diagnostic Issues

Bulimia nervosa is far more common in females than in males. Males are especially underrepresented in treatment-seeking samples, for reasons that have not yet been systematically examined.

Diagnostic Markers

No specific diagnostic test for bulimia nervosa currently exists. However, several laboratory abnormalities may occur as a consequence of purging and may increase diagnostic certainty. These include fluid and electrolyte abnormalities, such as hypokalemia (which can provoke cardiac arrhythmias), hypochloremia, and hyponatremia. The loss of gastric acid through vomiting may produce a metabolic alkalosis (elevated serum bicarbonate), and the frequent induction of diarrhea or dehydration through laxative and diuretic abuse can cause metabolic acidosis. Some individuals with bulimia nervosa exhibit mildly elevated levels of serum amylase, probably reflecting an increase in the salivary isoenzyme.

Physical examination usually yields no physical findings. However, inspection of the mouth may reveal significant and permanent loss of dental enamel, especially from lingual surfaces of the front teeth due to recurrent vomiting. These teeth may become chipped and appear ragged and "moth-eaten." There may also be an increased frequency of dental caries. In some individuals, the salivary glands, particularly the parotid glands, may become notably enlarged. Individuals who induce vomiting by manually stimulating the gag reflex may develop calluses or scars on the dorsal surface of the hand from repeated contact with the teeth. Serious cardiac and skeletal myopathies have been reported among individuals following repeated use of syrup of ipecac to induce vomiting.

Suicide Risk

Suicide risk is elevated in bulimia nervosa. Comprehensive evaluation of individuals with this disorder should include assessment of suicide-related ideation and behaviors as well as other risk factors for suicide, including a history of suicide attempts.

Functional Consequences of Bulimia Nervosa

Individuals with bulimia nervosa may exhibit a range of functional limitations associated with the disorder. A minority of individuals report severe role impairment, with the social-life domain most likely to be adversely affected by bulimia nervosa.

Differential Diagnosis

Anorexia nervosa, binge-eating/purging type. Individuals whose binge-eating behavior occurs only during episodes of anorexia nervosa are given the diagnosis anorexia nervosa, binge-eating/purging type, and should not be given the additional diagnosis of bulimia nervosa. For individuals with an initial diagnosis of anorexia nervosa who binge and purge but whose presentation no longer meets the full criteria for anorexia nervosa, binge-eating/purging type (e.g., when weight is normal), a diagnosis of bulimia nervosa should be given only when all criteria for bulimia nervosa have been met for at least 3 months.

Binge-eating disorder. Some individuals binge eat but do not engage in regular inappropriate compensatory behaviors. In these cases, the diagnosis of binge-eating disorder should be considered.

Kleine-Levin syndrome. In certain neurological or other medical conditions, such as Kleine-Levin syndrome, there is disturbed eating behavior, but the characteristic psychological features of bulimia nervosa, such as overconcern with body shape and weight, are not present.

Major depressive disorder, with atypical features. Overeating is common in major depressive disorder, with atypical features, but individuals with this disorder do not engage in inappropriate compensatory behaviors and do not exhibit the excessive concern with body shape and weight characteristic of bulimia nervosa. If criteria for both disorders are met, both diagnoses should be given.

Borderline personality disorder. Binge-eating behavior is included in the impulsive behavior criterion that is part of the definition of borderline personality disorder. If the criteria for both borderline personality disorder and bulimia nervosa are met, both diagnoses should be given.

Comorbidity

Comorbidity with mental disorders is common in individuals with bulimia nervosa, with most experiencing at least one other mental disorder and many experiencing multiple comorbidities. Comorbidity is not limited to any particular subset but rather occurs across a wide range of mental disorders. There is an increased frequency of depressive symptoms (e.g., low self-esteem) and bipolar and depressive disorders (particularly depressive disorders) in individuals with bulimia nervosa. In many individuals, the mood disturbance begins at the same time as or following the development of bulimia nervosa, and individuals often ascribe their mood disturbances to the bulimia nervosa. However, in some individuals, the mood disturbance clearly precedes the development of bulimia nervosa. There may also be an increased frequency of anxiety symptoms (e.g., fear of social situations) or anxiety disorders. These mood and anxiety disturbances frequently remit following effective treatment of the bulimia nervosa. The lifetime prevalence of substance use, particularly alcohol or stimulant use, is at least 30% among individuals with bulimia nervosa. Stimulant use often begins in an attempt to control appetite and weight. A substantial percentage of individuals with bulimia nervosa also have personality features that meet criteria for one or more personality disorders, most frequently borderline personality disorder.

Binge-Eating Disorder

Diagnostic Criteria	307.51 (F50.8)

A. Recurrent episodes of binge eating. An episode of binge eating is characterized by both of the following:

1. Eating, in a discrete period of time (e.g., within any 2-hour period), an amount of food that is definitely larger than what most people would eat in a similar period of time under similar circumstances.
2. A sense of lack of control over eating during the episode (e.g., a feeling that one cannot stop eating or control what or how much one is eating).

B. The binge-eating episodes are associated with three (or more) of the following:

1. Eating much more rapidly than normal.
2. Eating until feeling uncomfortably full.
3. Eating large amounts of food when not feeling physically hungry.
4. Eating alone because of feeling embarrassed by how much one is eating.
5. Feeling disgusted with oneself, depressed, or very guilty afterward.

C. Marked distress regarding binge eating is present.
D. The binge eating occurs, on average, at least once a week for 3 months.
E. The binge eating is not associated with the recurrent use of inappropriate compensatory behavior as in bulimia nervosa and does not occur exclusively during the course of bulimia nervosa or anorexia nervosa.

Specify if:

In partial remission: After full criteria for binge-eating disorder were previously met, binge eating occurs at an average frequency of less than one episode per week for a sustained period of time.

In full remission: After full criteria for binge-eating disorder were previously met, none of the criteria have been met for a sustained period of time.

Specify current severity:
The minimum level of severity is based on the frequency of episodes of binge eating (see below). The level of severity may be increased to reflect other symptoms and the degree of functional disability.

Mild: 1–3 binge-eating episodes per week.
Moderate: 4–7 binge-eating episodes per week.
Severe: 8–13 binge-eating episodes per week.
Extreme: 14 or more binge-eating episodes per week.

Diagnostic Features

The essential feature of binge-eating disorder is recurrent episodes of binge eating that must occur, on average, at least once per week for 3 months (Criterion D). An "episode of binge eating" is defined as eating, in a discrete period of time, an amount of food that is definitely larger than most people would eat in a similar period of time under similar circumstances (Criterion A1). The context in which the eating occurs may affect the clinician's estimation of whether the intake is excessive. For example, a quantity of food that might be regarded as excessive for a typical meal might be considered normal during a celebration or holiday meal. A "discrete period of time" refers to a limited period, usually less than 2 hours. A single episode of binge eating need not be restricted to one setting. For example, an individual may begin a binge in a restaurant and then continue to eat on returning home. Continual snacking on small amounts of food throughout the day would not be considered an eating binge.

An occurrence of excessive food consumption must be accompanied by a sense of lack of control (Criterion A2) to be considered an episode of binge eating. An indicator of loss of control is the inability to refrain from eating or to stop eating once started. Some individuals describe a dissociative quality during, or following, the binge-eating episodes. The impairment in control associated with binge eating may not be absolute; for example, an individual may continue binge eating while the telephone is ringing but will cease if a roommate or spouse unexpectedly enters the room. Some individuals report that their binge-eating episodes are no longer characterized by an acute feeling of loss of control but rather by a more generalized pattern of uncontrolled eating. If individuals report that they have abandoned efforts to control their eating, loss of control may still be considered as present. Binge eating can also be planned in some instances.

The type of food consumed during binges varies both across individuals and for a given individual. Binge eating appears to be characterized more by an abnormality in the amount of food consumed than by a craving for a specific nutrient.

Binge eating must be characterized by marked distress (Criterion C) and at least three of the following features: eating much more rapidly than normal; eating until feeling uncomfortably full; eating large amounts of food when not feeling physically hungry; eating alone because of feeling embarrassed by how much one is eating; and feeling disgusted with oneself, depressed, or very guilty afterward (Criterion B).

Individuals with binge-eating disorder are typically ashamed of their eating problems and attempt to conceal their symptoms. Binge eating usually occurs in secrecy or as inconspicuously as possible. The most common antecedent of binge eating is negative affect. Other triggers include interpersonal stressors; dietary restraint; negative feelings related to body weight, body shape, and food; and boredom. Binge eating may minimize or mitigate factors that precipitated the episode in the short-term, but negative self-evaluation and dysphoria often are the delayed consequences.

Associated Features Supporting Diagnosis

Binge-eating disorder occurs in normal-weight/overweight and obese individuals. It is reliably associated with overweight and obesity in treatment-seeking individuals. Nevertheless, binge-eating disorder is distinct from obesity. Most obese individuals do not engage in recurrent binge eating. In addition, compared with weight-matched obese individuals without binge-eating disorder, those with the disorder consume more calories in laboratory studies of eating behavior and have greater functional impairment, lower quality of life, more subjective distress, and greater psychiatric comorbidity.

Prevalence

Twelve-month prevalence of binge-eating disorder among U.S. adult (age 18 or older) females and males is 1.6% and 0.8%, respectively. The gender ratio is far less skewed in binge-eating disorder than in bulimia nervosa. Binge-eating disorder is as prevalent among females from racial or ethnic minority groups as has been reported for white females. The disorder is more prevalent among individuals seeking weight-loss treatment than in the general population.

Development and Course

Little is known about the development of binge-eating disorder. Both binge eating and loss-of-control eating without objectively excessive consumption occur in children and are associated with increased body fat, weight gain, and increases in psychological symptoms. Binge eating is common in adolescent and college-age samples. Loss-of-control eating or episodic binge eating may represent a prodromal phase of eating disorders for some individuals.

Dieting follows the development of binge eating in many individuals with binge-eating disorder. (This is in contrast to bulimia nervosa, in which dysfunctional dieting usually precedes the onset of binge eating.) Binge-eating disorder typically begins in adolescence or young adulthood but can begin in later adulthood. Individuals with binge-eating disorder who seek treatment usually are older than individuals with either bulimia nervosa or anorexia nervosa who seek treatment.

Remission rates in both natural course and treatment outcome studies are higher for binge-eating disorder than for bulimia nervosa or anorexia nervosa. Binge-eating disorder appears to be relatively persistent, and the course is comparable to that of bulimia nervosa in terms of severity and duration. Crossover from binge-eating disorder to other eating disorders is uncommon.

Risk and Prognostic Factors

Genetic and physiological.   Binge-eating disorder appears to run in families, which may reflect additive genetic influences.

Culture-Related Diagnostic Issues

Binge-eating disorder occurs with roughly similar frequencies in most industrialized countries, including the United States, Canada, many European countries, Australia, and New Zealand. In the United States, the prevalence of binge-eating disorder appears comparable among non-Latino whites, Latinos, Asians, and African Americans.

Functional Consequences of Binge-Eating Disorder

Binge-eating disorder is associated with a range of functional consequences, including social role adjustment problems, impaired health-related quality of life and life satisfaction, increased medical morbidity and mortality, and associated increased health care utilization compared with body mass index (BMI)–matched control subjects. It may also be associated with an increased risk for weight gain and the development of obesity.

Differential Diagnosis

Bulimia nervosa. Binge-eating disorder has recurrent binge eating in common with bulimia nervosa but differs from the latter disorder in some fundamental respects. In terms of clinical presentation, the recurrent inappropriate compensatory behavior (e.g., purging, driven exercise) seen in bulimia nervosa is absent in binge-eating disorder. Unlike individuals with bulimia nervosa, individuals with binge-eating disorder typically do not show marked or sustained dietary restriction designed to influence body weight and shape between binge-eating episodes. They may, however, report frequent attempts at dieting. Binge-eating disorder also differs from bulimia nervosa in terms of response to treatment. Rates of improvement are consistently higher among individuals with binge-eating disorder than among those with bulimia nervosa.

Obesity. Binge-eating disorder is associated with overweight and obesity but has several key features that are distinct from obesity. First, levels of overvaluation of body weight and shape are higher in obese individuals with the disorder than in those without the disorder. Second, rates of psychiatric comorbidity are significantly higher among obese individuals with the disorder compared with those without the disorder. Third, the long-term successful outcome of evidence-based psychological treatments for binge-eating disorder can be contrasted with the absence of effective long-term treatments for obesity.

Bipolar and depressive disorders. Increases in appetite and weight gain are included in the criteria for major depressive episode and in the atypical features specifiers for depressive and bipolar disorders. Increased eating in the context of a major depressive episode may or may not be associated with loss of control. If the full criteria for both disorders are met, both diagnoses can be given. Binge eating and other symptoms of disordered eating are seen in association with bipolar disorder. If the full criteria for both disorders are met, both diagnoses should be given.

Borderline personality disorder. Binge eating is included in the impulsive behavior criterion that is part of the definition of borderline personality disorder. If the full criteria for both disorders are met, both diagnoses should be given.

Comorbidity

Binge-eating disorder is associated with significant psychiatric comorbidity that is comparable to that of bulimia nervosa and anorexia nervosa. The most common comorbid disorders are bipolar disorders, depressive disorders, anxiety disorders, and, to a lesser degree, substance use disorders. The psychiatric comorbidity is linked to the severity of binge eating and not to the degree of obesity.

Other Specified Feeding or Eating Disorder

307.59 (F50.8)

This category applies to presentations in which symptoms characteristic of a feeding and eating disorder that cause clinically significant distress or impairment in social, occupational, or other important areas of functioning predominate but do not meet the full criteria for any of the disorders in the feeding and eating disorders diagnostic class. The other specified feeding or eating disorder category is used in situations in which the clinician chooses to communicate the specific reason that the presentation does not meet the criteria for any specific feeding and eating disorder. This is done by recording "other specified feeding or eating disorder" followed by the specific reason (e.g., "bulimia nervosa of low frequency").

Examples of presentations that can be specified using the "other specified" designation include the following:

1. **Atypical anorexia nervosa:** All of the criteria for anorexia nervosa are met, except that despite significant weight loss, the individual's weight is within or above the normal range.

2. **Bulimia nervosa (of low frequency and/or limited duration):** All of the criteria for bulimia nervosa are met, except that the binge eating and inappropriate compensatory behaviors occur, on average, less than once a week and/or for less than 3 months.

3. **Binge-eating disorder (of low frequency and/or limited duration):** All of the criteria for binge-eating disorder are met, except that the binge eating occurs, on average, less than once a week and/or for less than 3 months.

4. **Purging disorder:** Recurrent purging behavior to influence weight or shape (e.g., self-induced vomiting; misuse of laxatives, diuretics, or other medications) in the absence of binge eating.

5. **Night eating syndrome:** Recurrent episodes of night eating, as manifested by eating after awakening from sleep or by excessive food consumption after the evening meal. There is awareness and recall of the eating. The night eating is not better explained by external influences such as changes in the individual's sleep-wake cycle or by local social norms. The night eating causes significant distress and/or impairment in functioning. The disordered pattern of eating is not better explained by binge-eating disorder or another mental disorder, including substance use, and is not attributable to another medical disorder or to an effect of medication.

Unspecified Feeding or Eating Disorder

307.50 (F50.9)

This category applies to presentations in which symptoms characteristic of a feeding and eating disorder that cause clinically significant distress or impairment in social, occupational, or other important areas of functioning predominate but do not meet the full criteria for any of the disorders in the feeding and eating disorders diagnostic class. The unspecified feeding or eating disorder category is used in situations in which the clinician chooses *not* to specify the reason that the criteria are not met for a specific feeding and eating disorder, and includes presentations in which there is insufficient information to make a more specific diagnosis (e.g., in emergency room settings).

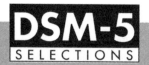

Feeding and Eating Disorders

DSM-5® Guidebook

307.52 (F__.__) Pica
307.53 (F98.21) Rumination Disorder
307.59 (F50.8) Avoidant/Restrictive Food Intake Disorder
307.1 (F50.0_) Anorexia Nervosa
307.51 (F50.2) Bulimia Nervosa
307.51 (F50.8) Binge-Eating Disorder
307.59 (F50.8) Other Specified Feeding or Eating Disorder
307.50 (F50.9) Unspecified Feeding or Eating Disorder

The chapter on feeding and eating disorders has combined the feeding disorders (pica, rumination disorder) from the DSM-IV chapter "Disorders Usually First Diagnosed in Infancy, Childhood, or Adolescence" with the eating disorders (anorexia nervosa, bulimia nervosa) to better reflect their shared phenomenology and pathophysiology. The diagnosis avoidant/restrictive food intake disorder replaces and extends the DSM-IV diagnosis feeding disorder of infancy or early childhood. In addition, binge-eating disorder, previously included in DSM-IV's Appendix B, has now achieved full disorder status. Feeding and eating disorders reflect dysfunctional appetitive drive and behavior and can span the entire age range. Table 1 lists the disorders included in this chapter.

TABLE 1. DSM-5 feeding and eating disorders

Pica

Rumination disorder

Avoidant/restrictive food intake disorder

Anorexia nervosa

Bulimia nervosa

Binge-eating disorder

Other specified feeding or eating disorder

Unspecified feeding or eating disorder

Disordered eating and eating-related behaviors have been recognized for centuries. Richard Morton (1636–1698) is credited with making the first clinical description of anorexia nervosa in 1689, but it was Sir William Gull (1816–1890) who coined the term in the late nineteenth century. Gull's patients were mostly emaciated young women with amenorrhea, constipation, and an abnormally slow pulse who were nonetheless remarkably overactive. His account of the disorder remains noteworthy for its attention to detail.

Despite Gull's and other descriptions, eating and feeding disorders were not listed in DSM until DSM-III, when they were included in the chapter "Disorders Usually First Diagnosed in Infancy, Childhood, or Adolescence." Eating disorders were given their own chapter in DSM-IV because it was clear that they could occur across the age range. In revisiting the issue, the DSM-5 Eating Disorders Work Group recommended that feeding disorders also be included in the same chapter with eating disorders because they, too, can occur across the age range.

Pica

The essential feature of pica is the eating of nonnutritive nonfood substances on a persistent basis for a period of at least 1 month. Medical accounts that resemble the modern-day definition of pica date back many centuries. Historically, pica has been considered either as an accompaniment to conditions such as pregnancy or developmental disabilities or as a symptom of medical disorders such as iron deficiency. Children up to age 24 months frequently mouth or even eat nonnutritive items, but this behavior does not suggest that the child has pica. Although frequently associated with children with developmental delays, pica is not confined to children or to individuals with intellectual developmental disorders.

Pica has been regarded as an independent disorder since its inclusion in DSM-III. The criteria were revised for DSM-5 to ensure that they can be used with individuals of any age.

Diagnostic Criteria for Pica

A. Persistent eating of nonnutritive, nonfood substances over a period of at least 1 month.
B. The eating of nonnutritive, nonfood substances is inappropriate to the developmental level of the individual.
C. The eating behavior is not part of a culturally supported or socially normative practice.
D. If the eating behavior occurs in the context of another mental disorder (e.g., intellectual disability [intellectual developmental disorder], autism spectrum disorder, schizophrenia) or medical condition (including pregnancy), it is sufficiently severe to warrant additional clinical attention.

Coding note: The ICD-9-CM code for pica is **307.52** and is used for children or adults. The ICD-10-CM codes for pica are **(F98.3)** in children and **(F50.8)** in adults.

Specify if:

In remission: After full criteria for pica were previously met, the criteria have not been met for a sustained period of time.

Criterion A

A single ingestion of a nonnutritive, nonfood substance is not sufficient to merit the diagnosis of pica. The eating must be persistent over a 1-month period. Changes to DSM-5 include the addition of the term *nonfood*; the wording "nonnutritive substances" was potentially problematic because, with nonfood not specified, the term could include foodstuffs with no nutritional value, such as diet soda.

Criterion B

Mouthing of objects, including nonnutritive, nonfood substances, is developmentally normal in young infants. A minimum age of 2 years is recommended because pica is not an appropriate diagnosis for young children.

Criterion C

People around the world eat clay or dirt (called *geophagy*) for a variety of reasons. Commonly, geophagy is a traditional cultural activity that takes place during pregnancy, for religious ceremonies, or as a remedy for disease, particularly in Central Africa and the Southern United States. The indigenous Pomo of Northern California also include dirt in their diet. Although it is a cultural practice, it may also fill a physiological need (or perceived need) for nutrients.

Criterion D

Pica frequently occurs in individuals with developmental delays and sometimes in pregnant women. Individuals with schizophrenia may have delusional beliefs about the need to ingest nonfood substances. If the eating behavior is severe enough to warrant independent clinical attention, then the additional diagnosis of pica is appropriate. DSM-5 has changed the wording from "during the course of" to "in the context of" to retain consistency with parallel criteria for rumination disorder and avoidant/restrictive food intake disorder, and because the example given (intellectual developmental disorder) does not run a course.

Rumination Disorder

Rumination disorder is characterized by the repeated regurgitation of food. Included in some form in the medical literature from the seventeenth century onward, rumination disorder occurs across the age range and in both genders. Individuals with this disorder repeatedly regurgitate swallowed or partially digested food, which may then be rechewed and either reswallowed or expelled. Adolescents and adults may be less likely to rechew regurgitated material. There is no involuntary retching, nausea, heartburn, odors, or abdominal pains associated with the regurgitation, as there is with typical vomiting. Although the disorder occurs more commonly in infants, young children, and individuals with developmental disabilities, it also occurs in otherwise healthy adolescents and adults. Unlike in typical vomiting, the regurgitation is typically described as effortless and unforced.

DSM-III included rumination disorder of infancy as an independent disorder. The criteria have been modified for DSM-5 to ensure that they are appropriate for individuals of any age.

Diagnostic Criteria for Rumination Disorder   **307.53 (F98.21)**

A. Repeated regurgitation of food over a period of at least 1 month. Regurgitated food may be re-chewed, re-swallowed, or spit out.

B. The repeated regurgitation is not attributable to an associated gastrointestinal or other medical condition (e.g., gastroesophageal reflux, pyloric stenosis).

C. The eating disturbance does not occur exclusively during the course of anorexia nervosa, bulimia nervosa, binge-eating disorder, or avoidant/restrictive food intake disorder.

D. If the symptoms occur in the context of another mental disorder (e.g., intellectual disability [intellectual developmental disorder] or another neurodevelopmental disorder), they are sufficiently severe to warrant additional clinical attention.

Specify if:

In remission: After full criteria for rumination disorder were previously met, the criteria have not been met for a sustained period of time.

Criterion A

This criterion requires repeated regurgitation of food for at least 1 month. Not all individuals with rumination disorder, particularly older individuals and those with normal intelligence, rechew the regurgitated food. Therefore, DSM-5 has deleted the rechewing requirement and instead states, "Regurgitated food may be re-chewed, re-swallowed, or spit out." In addition, the DSM-IV requirement that the behavior follow "a period of normal functioning" has been deleted because this may be difficult to determine.

Criterion B

Individuals with rumination disorder may have a history of reflux, and it may be difficult clinically to reliably parse out the medical and psychological components of the behavior. In recognition of this clinical difficulty, DSM-5 requires ruling out an associated gastrointestinal or other medical condition.

Criterion C

Rumination behavior is well documented to occur in persons with conventional eating disorders. This criterion requires that the rumination be more than a symptom of one of the eating disorders. If it occurs apart from the eating disorder, then it can be independently diagnosed.

Criterion D

Rumination disorder commonly occurs in the context of developmental delays, often as a means of self-stimulation. In these cases, this behavior is more appropriately considered a symptom of these other disorders or conditions. If the rumination behavior is severe enough to warrant independent clinical attention, then the additional diagnosis of rumination disorder is appropriate. DSM-5 has changed the wording from "during the course of" to "in the context of" to maintain consistency with parallel criteria for pica and avoidant/restrictive food intake disorder and because the example given (intellectual disability [intellectual developmental disorder]) does not, strictly speaking, run a course.

Avoidant/Restrictive Food Intake Disorder

Avoidant/restrictive food intake disorder replaces and extends feeding disorder of infancy or early childhood from DSM-IV. This disorder is a disturbance of eating or feeding behavior that takes the form of avoiding or restricting food intake. The change in the formal name of the disorder reflects the fact that there are a number of types of presentation that occur across the age range rather than being restricted to infancy and early childhood. Three main subtypes have been identified in the existing literature: individuals who do not eat enough or show little interest in feeding or eating; individuals who accept only a limited diet in relation to sensory features; and individuals whose food refusal is related to aversive experience.

Avoidance or restriction associated with insufficient intake or lack of interest in food usually develops in infancy or early childhood, although it can begin in adolescence; onset in adulthood is rare. This disorder does not include developmentally normal food avoidance, which is characterized by picky eating in childhood or reduced food intake associated with advanced age. Pregnant women may restrict intake or avoid certain foods because of altered sensory sensitivities, but this is a self-limited behavior and the diagnosis of avoidant/restrictive food intake disorder is not warranted unless the eating disturbance is extreme and full criteria are met.

Avoidant/restrictive food intake disorder appears equally common in males and females in infancy and childhood. Various functional consequences are associated with this disorder: impairments in physical development, relationship and social difficulties, caregiver stress, and problems in family functioning.

This diagnosis has been renamed from feeding disorder of infancy or early childhood in DSM-IV, a diagnosis that was rarely used. In revamping this category, the authors of DSM-5 expect that the new category will be more useful. The category should potentially fill a clinical need because a substantial number of individuals—not exclusively children and adolescents—restrict their food intake and develop significant physiological and/or psychosocial problems, but their presentations fail to meet criteria for an eating disorder. Avoidance/restrictive food intake disorder is a broad category intended to capture this range of presentations.

Diagnostic Criteria for Avoidant/Restrictive
Food Intake Disorder   307.59 (F50.8)

A. An eating or feeding disturbance (e.g., apparent lack of interest in eating or food; avoidance based on the sensory characteristics of food; concern about aversive consequences of eating) as manifested by persistent failure to meet appropriate nutritional and/or energy needs associated with one (or more) of the following:

1. Significant weight loss (or failure to achieve expected weight gain or faltering growth in children).
2. Significant nutritional deficiency.
3. Dependence on enteral feeding or oral nutritional supplements.
4. Marked interference with psychosocial functioning.

B. The disturbance is not better explained by lack of available food or by an associated culturally sanctioned practice.

C. The eating disturbance does not occur exclusively during the course of anorexia nervosa or bulimia nervosa, and there is no evidence of a disturbance in the way in which one's body weight or shape is experienced.

D. The eating disturbance is not attributable to a concurrent medical condition or not better explained by another mental disorder. When the eating disturbance occurs in the context of another condition or disorder, the severity of the eating disturbance exceeds that routinely associated with the condition or disorder and warrants additional clinical attention.

Specify if:

In remission: After full criteria for avoidant/restrictive food intake disorder were previously met, the criteria have not been met for a sustained period of time.

Criterion A

Many young children with avoidant/restrictive food intake difficulties had symptoms that failed to meet DSM-IV criteria for feeding disorder because of the primary focus in those criteria on failure to gain weight or weight loss, as well as the fact that certain features of presentation are also commonly seen in older individuals. "Feeding disturbance" has been replaced by "an eating or feeding disturbance" to account for the wider age range of people who have this disorder. Consequences resulting from food avoidance or restriction may persist, and this criterion has been expanded beyond weight loss or inability to gain weight. Faltering growth, nutritional deficiency, or dependency on enteral feeding or oral nutritional supplements, and marked interference with psychosocial functioning have been added because these are common clinically significant consequences of such eating or feeding disturbances.

Criterion B

Because extreme poverty and cultural practices, such as religious fasting, can also result in significant weight loss, this criterion includes the phrase "not better explained by lack of available food" and the requirement that there be no evidence that a "culturally sanctioned" practice alone, such as particular religious or cultural observations, might account for the disorder.

Criterion C

Restriction of energy intake relative to requirements resulting in weight loss is a core feature of anorexia nervosa and may be a compensatory behavior in bulimia nervosa. For older children or young adolescents, these disorders share a number of features, such as low weight and food avoidance. Anorexia nervosa, however, is associated with fear of gaining weight and perceptual disturbances regarding one's body weight or shape. In the case of bulimia nervosa, the restriction or fasting is a compensatory behavior for the recurrent episodes of binge eating. It is necessary to make a distinction between restricted food intake in the context of eating disorders, in which there are weight or shape concerns, and restricted food intake in which such concerns are not present.

Criterion D

Gastrointestinal (e.g., gastroesophageal reflux), endocrinological (e.g., diabetes), and neurological (e.g., those related to oral/esophageal/pharyngeal structural or functional problems) conditions can cause feeding disturbances and need to be distinguished from avoidant/restrictive food intake disorder.

Anorexia Nervosa

Anorexia nervosa is characterized by persistent energy intake restriction, an intense fear of gaining weight, and a distorted body self-perception. Anorexia nervosa was the first eating disorder described and appears to have been present at different points in history and to be present throughout different cultures. The disorder is associated with distorted self-image and other cognitive distortions regarding food and eating. Individuals with anorexia nervosa sometimes engage in repeated weighing, measuring, and assessing of their body in the mirror. The key clinical feature is defined as a refusal to maintain body weight at or above a minimally normal level for age, sex, developmental trajectory, and physical health. Anorexia nervosa is associated with high rates of morbidity (e.g., cardiac arrhythmias, growth retardation, osteoporosis) and mortality.

Anorexia nervosa typically has an onset in adolescence and is more prevalent among females. The disorder can affect men and women of any age, race or ethnicity, and socioeconomic background. The disorder has an estimated prevalence of 0.3%–1% in women and 0.1% in men.

Anorexia nervosa was listed in DSM-I as an example of psychophysiological gastrointestinal reaction and in DSM-II as a feeding disturbance within the special symptoms category. It finally achieved full disorder status in DSM-III. The core diagnostic criteria for anorexia nervosa are conceptually unchanged from DSM-IV, with one exception: *the requirement for amenorrhea has been eliminated* (DSM-IV's Criterion D). Some individuals with anorexia nervosa may exhibit all other symptoms and signs of the disorder and report at least some menstrual activity. In addition, this criterion could not be applied to premenarcheal girls, women taking oral contraceptives, post-menopausal women, or males. Because some data indicate that women who endorse amenorrhea have poorer bone health than do women who fail to meet this criterion, the information is clinically important even if not required for the diagnosis. In addition, the clinical characteristics and course for women with presentations that meet all the DSM-IV criteria for anorexia nervosa except amenorrhea closely resemble the characteristics of women with presentations that meet all of the criteria.

Diagnostic Criteria for Anorexia Nervosa

A. Restriction of energy intake relative to requirements, leading to a significantly low body weight in the context of age, sex, developmental trajectory, and physical health. *Significantly low weight* is defined as a weight that is less than minimally normal or, for children and adolescents, less than that minimally expected.

B. Intense fear of gaining weight or of becoming fat, or persistent behavior that interferes with weight gain, even though at a significantly low weight.

C. Disturbance in the way in which one's body weight or shape is experienced, undue influence of body weight or shape on self-evaluation, or persistent lack of recognition of the seriousness of the current low body weight.

Coding note: The ICD-9-CM code for anorexia nervosa is **307.1,** which is assigned regardless of the subtype. The ICD-10-CM code depends on the subtype (see below).

Specify whether:

(F50.01) Restricting type: During the last 3 months, the individual has not engaged in recurrent episodes of binge eating or purging behavior (i.e., self-induced vomiting or the misuse of laxatives, diuretics, or enemas). This subtype describes presentations in which weight loss is accomplished primarily through dieting, fasting, and/or excessive exercise.

(F50.02) Binge-eating/purging type: During the last 3 months, the individual has engaged in recurrent episodes of binge eating or purging behavior (i.e., self-induced vomiting or the misuse of laxatives, diuretics, or enemas).

Specify if:

In partial remission: After full criteria for anorexia nervosa were previously met, Criterion A (low body weight) has not been met for a sustained period, but either Criterion B (intense fear of gaining weight or becoming fat or behavior that interferes with weight gain) or Criterion C (disturbances in self-perception of weight and shape) is still met.

In full remission: After full criteria for anorexia nervosa were previously met, none of the criteria have been met for a sustained period of time.

Specify current severity:

The minimum level of severity is based, for adults, on current body mass index (BMI) (see below) or, for children and adolescents, on BMI percentile. The ranges below are derived from World Health Organization categories for thinness in adults; for children and adolescents, corresponding BMI percentiles should be used. The level of severity may be increased to reflect clinical symptoms, the degree of functional disability, and the need for supervision.

Mild: BMI $\geq$ 17 kg/m^2
Moderate: BMI 16–16.99 kg/m^2
Severe: BMI 15–15.99 kg/m^2
Extreme: BMI < 15 kg/m^2

Criterion A

The DSM-IV wording "Refusal to maintain body weight at or above a minimally normal weight for age and height" has been changed to emphasize the importance of energy homeostasis for maintenance of a minimally normal weight. This change allows for applicability of the diagnosis to individuals who employ increased activity as a means of reducing weight.

Criterion B

DSM-IV required "fear of weight gain." A significant minority of individuals with anorexia nervosa, however, explicitly deny experiencing such fear. Therefore, DSM-5 has added a clause to focus on behavior, "persistent behavior that interferes with weight gain, even though at a significantly low weight."

Criterion C

The wording of this item has changed from "denial of the seriousness of the current low body weight" in DSM-IV to "persistent lack of recognition of the seriousness of the current low body weight." The word *denial* was removed because of the lack of empirical evidence supporting its use and the concern that it conveyed a paternalistic and pejorative attitude.

Subtypes and Specifiers

In DSM-5, the subtypes restricting and binge-eating/purging are specified for the last 3 months. Although data suggest that subtyping is useful clinically and for research purposes, there is significant crossover between subtypes, and clinicians had difficulty specifying the subtype for the "current episode" of illness (the DSM-IV standard).

Clinicians can also specify whether the person's disorder is in full remission or in partial remission. The distinction is that with partial remission, in which low body weight (Criterion A) is no longer an issue, the person still has an intense fear of gaining weight or of being fat, or has a disturbed body image.

Current severity can be indicated by specifying whether the disorder is mild, moderate, severe, or extreme, based on BMI.

Bulimia Nervosa

Bulimia nervosa is characterized by episodes of bingeing on food (i.e., consuming a large amount of food in a short amount of time), followed by attempts to purge the body of the food via vomiting, laxatives, or excessive exercise. The behavior is performed in the context of overconcern with weight and shape. Russell (1979) observed that both anorexia nervosa and bulimia nervosa are developmental disorders that share the characteristics fear of fatness and body image distortion. As with anorexia nervosa, there are medical consequences of bulimia nervosa, including loss of electrolytes, erosion of tooth enamel (due to repeated exposure to acidic gastric contents), cavities, stomach ulcers, stomach or esophagus ruptures, constipation, irregular heartbeat, and an increased tendency toward suicidal behavior. Bulimia nervosa also exhibits marked differences from anorexia nervosa. Individuals with bulimia nervosa tend to develop eating disorder symptoms later in life, generally lose less weight, and have a tendency to be more extroverted and impulsive than persons with anorexia nervosa.

This disorder, simply called "bulimia," was included in DSM-III. The name was changed to bulimia nervosa in DSM-III-R. Approximately 90% of people diagnosed with bulimia nervosa are women, and its prevalence is estimated at 1.0%–1.5% in young women.

The only change in the criteria is a reduction in the required minimum average frequency of binge eating and inappropriate compensatory behavior (Criterion C). Clinicians can now rate severity levels that range from mild to extreme depending on the number of episodes of inappropriate compensatory behaviors per week.

Although DSM-IV required that subtype (purging or nonpurging) be specified, a literature review indicated that individuals with the nonpurging subtype closely resembled individuals with binge-eating disorder. In addition, precisely how to define nonpurging inappropriate behaviors (e.g., fasting or excessive exercise) was unclear. For these reasons, DSM-5 has eliminated the purging and nonpurging subtypes for bulimia nervosa. Instead, clinicians can specify whether the disorder is in partial or full remission and the current severity (mild, moderate, severe, extreme).

Diagnostic Criteria for Bulimia Nervosa   **307.51 (F50.2)**

A. Recurrent episodes of binge eating. An episode of binge eating is characterized by both of the following:

   1. Eating, in a discrete period of time (e.g., within any 2-hour period), an amount of food that is definitely larger than what most individuals would eat in a similar period of time under similar circumstances.

   2. A sense of lack of control over eating during the episode (e.g., a feeling that one cannot stop eating or control what or how much one is eating).

B. Recurrent inappropriate compensatory behaviors in order to prevent weight gain, such as self-induced vomiting; misuse of laxatives, diuretics, or other medications; fasting; or excessive exercise.

C. The binge eating and inappropriate compensatory behaviors both occur, on average, at least once a week for 3 months.

D. Self-evaluation is unduly influenced by body shape and weight.

E. The disturbance does not occur exclusively during episodes of anorexia nervosa.

Specify if:

   In partial remission: After full criteria for bulimia nervosa were previously met, some, but not all, of the criteria have been met for a sustained period of time.

In full remission: After full criteria for bulimia nervosa were previously met, none of the criteria have been met for a sustained period of time.

Specify current severity:

The minimum level of severity is based on the frequency of inappropriate compensatory behaviors (see below). The level of severity may be increased to reflect other symptoms and the degree of functional disability.

Mild: An average of 1–3 episodes of inappropriate compensatory behaviors per week.

Moderate: An average of 4–7 episodes of inappropriate compensatory behaviors per week.

Severe: An average of 8–13 episodes of inappropriate compensatory behaviors per week.

Extreme: An average of 14 or more episodes of inappropriate compensatory behaviors per week.

Criterion A

Many people may experience an isolated episode of overeating, such as at a party with unlimited free food. Bulimia nervosa is an appropriate diagnosis in cases in which there are recurrent episodes of binge eating that occur during a discrete period of time and involve the consumption of a large amount of food, and the person reports feeling a lack of control.

Criterion B

The bulimia nervosa diagnosis requires that the binge eating be accompanied by recurrent inappropriate compensatory behaviors intended to counteract the effects of the binge episode and prevent weight gain (e.g., vomiting, laxative abuse, diuretic abuse, excessive exercise).

Criterion C

Although DSM-IV required that episodes of binge eating and inappropriate compensatory behaviors both occur, on average, twice per week over a 3-month period, research found that the clinical characteristics of individuals reporting bingeing and purging once per week were similar to those of individuals whose behavior met the DSM-IV twice-per-week criterion. DSM-5 therefore requires that the binge eating and inappropriate compensatory behaviors occur at least once a week for 3 months.

Criterion D

Individuals with bulimia nervosa are preoccupied with body shape and weight. They may report low self-esteem due to body image issues.

Criterion E

Individuals with anorexia nervosa may have a presentation that falls under the subtype referred to as *binge-eating/purging type,* which must be differentiated from bulimia nervosa. The diagnosis of anorexia nervosa requires a refusal to maintain normal body weight. When that requirement is met, the appropriate diagnosis is anorexia nervosa.

Binge-Eating Disorder

Binge-eating disorder is characterized by recurrent episodes of binge eating without the recurrent use of compensatory behaviors. It was listed in Appendix B ("Criteria Sets and Axes Provided for Further Study") in DSM-IV, and the DSM-5 Eating Disorders Work Group recommended that it achieve full disorder status. Binge-eating disorder is the most frequent eating disorder in the United States (1.6% of women, 0.8% of men) and is more prevalent among those seeking weight loss treatment than in the general population.

The distinction between binge-eating disorder and bulimia nervosa is sometimes unclear, and the two categories may represent different stages of the same underlying disorder. Compared with individuals with bulimia nervosa, people with binge-eating disorder are generally older, are more likely to be male, and have a later age at onset of the disorder.

Approximately two-thirds of individuals with binge-eating disorder have a history of using inappropriate compensatory behaviors, suggesting a past diagnosis of bulimia nervosa. Although weight and shape concerns are not required for the diagnosis, they are commonly part of the presentation.

Clinicians can rate current severity based on number of binge-eating episodes per week (although the level of severity may be increased to reflect other symptoms and the degree of functional disability). Clinicians can also specify whether the disorder is in partial or full remission.

Diagnostic Criteria for Binge-Eating Disorder   307.51 (F50.8)

A. Recurrent episodes of binge eating. An episode of binge eating is characterized by both of the following:

  1. Eating, in a discrete period of time (e.g., within any 2-hour period), an amount of food that is definitely larger than what most people would eat in a similar period of time under similar circumstances.

  2. A sense of lack of control over eating during the episode (e.g., a feeling that one cannot stop eating or control what or how much one is eating).

B. The binge-eating episodes are associated with three (or more) of the following:

  1. Eating much more rapidly than normal.
  2. Eating until feeling uncomfortably full.
  3. Eating large amounts of food when not feeling physically hungry.
  4. Eating alone because of feeling embarrassed by how much one is eating.
  5. Feeling disgusted with oneself, depressed, or very guilty afterward.

C. Marked distress regarding binge eating is present.

D. The binge eating occurs, on average, at least once a week for 3 months.

E. The binge eating is not associated with the recurrent use of inappropriate compensatory behavior as in bulimia nervosa and does not occur exclusively during the course of bulimia nervosa or anorexia nervosa.

Specify if:

In partial remission: After full criteria for binge-eating disorder were previously met, binge eating occurs at an average frequency of less than one episode per week for a sustained period of time.

In full remission: After full criteria for binge-eating disorder were previously met, none of the criteria have been met for a sustained period of time.

Specify current severity:

The minimum level of severity is based on the frequency of episodes of binge eating (see below). The level of severity may be increased to reflect other symptoms and the degree of functional disability.

Mild: 1–3 binge-eating episodes per week.

Moderate: 4–7 binge-eating episodes per week.

Severe: 8–13 binge-eating episodes per week.

Extreme: 14 or more binge-eating episodes per week.

Criterion A

The requirement of binge eating mirrors that for bulimia nervosa. The criterion requires "recurrent episodes" to differentiate this disorder from context-specific instances where an individual may binge on food, such as at a wedding or banquet.

Criterion B

Criterion B requires at least three of five indicators of impaired control: eating much more rapidly than usual; eating until feeling uncomfortably full; eating large amounts of food when not hungry; eating alone because of embarrassment; and feeling disgust, depression, or guilt after the episode. The best overall indicators for correctly identifying binge eating are "eating large amounts of food when not feeling physically hungry" and "eating alone because of feeling embarrassed." Among men the most common feature of binge eating is eating more rapidly than usual, whereas among women the most common feature is feeling disgusted, depressed, or very guilty afterward. Research indicates that the requirement for three or more symptoms yields the most accurate prediction of binge eating while minimizing the false positives.

Criterion C

This criterion speaks to the specificity of distress associated with the binge eating. Distress related to co-occurring disorders would not meet this criterion.

Criterion D

Analyses based on once-weekly and twice-weekly classifications were remarkably similar. In DSM-IV Appendix B, it was suggested that the frequency of binge days, as opposed to binge episodes, be assessed, and that a minimum average frequency of twice per week over 6 months be required. Research indicates that criteria identical to those for bulimia nervosa would not change caseness significantly. Therefore, Criterion D was changed to be similar to Criterion C for bulimia nervosa, requiring at least once a week for 3 months.

Criterion E

Binge-eating disorder is characterized by the absence of recurrent use of inappropriate compensatory mechanisms after eating large amounts of food.

Other Specified Feeding or Eating Disorder and Unspecified Feeding or Eating Disorder

Other specified and unspecified feeding or eating disorder should be considered as diagnoses when the individual has symptoms of a feeding and eating disorder that are distressing and cause impairment but do not meet the full criteria for a more specific disorder in the class.

The categories replace DSM-IV's eating disorder not otherwise specified. The category other specified feeding or eating disorder is used when the clinician chooses to communicate the reason that the presentation does not meet full criteria. The clinician is encouraged to record the specific reason (e.g., atypical anorexia nervosa).

The category unspecified feeding or eating disorder is used when the clinician chooses not to specify the reason the criteria are not met, or there is insufficient information to make a more specific diagnosis.

Other Specified Feeding or Eating Disorder 307.59 (F50.8)

This category applies to presentations in which symptoms characteristic of a feeding and eating disorder that cause clinically significant distress or impairment in social, occupational, or other important areas of functioning predominate but do not meet the full criteria for any of the disorders in the feeding and eating disorders diagnostic class. The other specified feeding or eating disorder category is used in situations in which the clinician chooses to communicate the specific reason that the presentation does not meet the criteria for any specific feeding and eating disorder. This is done by recording "other specified feeding or eating disorder" followed by the specific reason (e.g., "bulimia nervosa of low frequency").

Examples of presentations that can be specified using the "other specified" designation include the following:

1. **Atypical anorexia nervosa:** All of the criteria for anorexia nervosa are met, except that despite significant weight loss, the individual's weight is within or above the normal range.
2. **Bulimia nervosa (of low frequency and/or limited duration):** All of the criteria for bulimia nervosa are met, except that the binge eating and inappropriate compensatory behaviors occur, on average, less than once a week and/or for less than 3 months.
3. **Binge-eating disorder (of low frequency and/or limited duration):** All of the criteria for binge-eating disorder are met, except that the binge eating occurs, on average, less than once a week and/or for less than 3 months.
4. **Purging disorder:** Recurrent purging behavior to influence weight or shape (e.g., self-induced vomiting; misuse of laxatives, diuretics, or other medications) in the absence of binge eating.

5. **Night eating syndrome:** Recurrent episodes of night eating, as manifested by eating after awakening from sleep or by excessive food consumption after the evening meal. There is awareness and recall of the eating. The night eating is not better explained by external influences such as changes in the individual's sleep-wake cycle or by local social norms. The night eating causes significant distress and/or impairment in functioning. The disordered pattern of eating is not better explained by binge-eating disorder or another mental disorder, including substance use, and is not attributable to another medical disorder or to an effect of medication.

Unspecified Feeding or Eating Disorder 307.50 (F50.9)

This category applies to presentations in which symptoms characteristic of a feeding and eating disorder that cause clinically significant distress or impairment in social, occupational, or other important areas of functioning predominate but do not meet the full criteria for any of the disorders in the feeding and eating disorders diagnostic class. The unspecified feeding or eating disorder category is used in situations in which the clinician chooses *not* to specify the reason that the criteria are not met for a specific feeding and eating disorder, and includes presentations in which there is insufficient information to make a more specific diagnosis (e.g., in emergency room settings).

KEY POINTS

- This chapter combines the feeding disorders, formerly placed in the DSM-IV chapter "Disorders Usually First Diagnosed in Infancy, Childhood, or Adolescence," with the eating disorders. Both groups of disorders are characterized by disturbed consummatory behaviors.

- The criteria for pica and rumination disorder have been revised to ensure that the disorders can be diagnosed in persons of all ages. Similarly, avoidant/restrictive food intake disorder no longer has an age restriction.

- The requirement that anorexia nervosa be accompanied by amenorrhea has been dropped because research showed little difference between those with or without the symptom.

- With bulimia nervosa, the only change in the criteria is a reduction in the required minimum average frequency of binge eating and inappropriate compensatory behavior to one episode per week (Criterion C), because research did not support the requirement in DSM-IV for two episodes per week.

- Binge-eating disorder has been elevated to full disorder status in DSM-5.

Reference

Russell G: Bulimia nervosa: an ominous variant of anorexia nervosa. Psychol Med 9:429–448, 1979

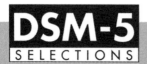

Feeding and Eating Disorders

DSM-5® Clinical Cases

Introduction

John W. Barnhill, M.D.

Until the publication of DSM-5, half of the people in eating disorder specialty clinics did not meet criteria for either of the two specific eating disorder categories—anorexia nervosa or bulimia nervosa—and instead received the nonspecific diagnosis of eating disorder not otherwise specified (EDNOS). This percentage swelled even further in general psychiatric outpatient settings. A large percentage of patients with impairment and distress related to eating problems were left, therefore, without a diagnosis that specifically described their condition.

DSM-5 has made multiple changes to help subdivide the eating disorder population into coherent and evidence-based subgroups. For example, binge-eating disorder (BED) has been moved out of the DSM-IV appendix that included criteria sets provided for further study and into the main body of the DSM-5 text. The criteria for anorexia nervosa (AN) remain conceptually unchanged but have been expanded in two ways. First, the requirement for amenorrhea has been eliminated. Second, a previous core AN criterion, the expressed fear of weight gain, is not always present in people who appear to display robust symptoms of AN; in order to remedy this quandary, DSM-5 adds an alternative to the "expressed fear" criterion: the individual may manifest persistent behavior that interferes with weight gain. This alternative criterion allows the diagnosis of people whose behavior is indicative of AN but who have impaired insight, suboptimal levels of cooperation or transparency, or alternative rationales for food restriction. Bulimia nervosa (BN) also stays conceptually the same in DSM-5, but the threshold for diagnosis has been lowered by reducing the frequency of binge eating and compensatory behavior from twice to once weekly.

Avoidant/restrictive food intake disorder (ARFID) is a new DSM-5 diagnosis that describes people who restrict or avoid food in a way that leads to significant impairment but who do not meet criteria for AN. A broad and inclusive category, ARFID includes individuals who previously met criteria for the DSM-IV diagnosis feeding disorder of infancy or early childhood. ARFID describes a cluster of patients who are generally children and adolescents but who can be any age.

By adding BED to the main text, reducing the threshold for a diagnosis of AN and BN, and creating the ARFID diagnosis, DSM-5 intends to more clearly describe subpopulations of patients who would previously have been recognized as having an eating disorder causing impairment but would have been characterized within the uninformative category of EDNOS. Furthermore, evidence indicates that individuals who meet the more flexible criteria are, in meaningful ways, similar to those who meet the older criteria. Controversy centers on whether this loosening and expansion of eating disorder diagnoses leads to assigning diagnoses to normal individuals; as is the case throughout DSM-5, diagnostic criteria require significant distress and/or impairment. Individuals within a normal range of eating behaviors should not receive a diagnosis.

Many patients with clinically relevant eating problems do not meet full criteria for a specific eating disorder. For example, an individual may meet all criteria for AN—including significant weight loss—but remain at a normal or above-normal weight. Such a presentation would warrant a diagnosis of specific eating disorder (atypical anorexia nervosa). Other specific eating disorders include bulimia or binge eating of low frequency or duration; purging without binge eating; and night eating syndrome. Finally, the diagnosis "unspecified feeding or eating disorder" is intended to describe individuals who have an apparent eating disorder but do not meet full criteria for a specific disorder, perhaps because of an inadequate amount of confirmatory information (e.g., in an emergency room setting).

In addition to disorders mentioned above, this chapter describes two feeding and eating disorders that are usually, but not always, diagnosed in childhood and adolescence: pica and rumination disorder. Pica refers to the persistent, clinically significant eating of nonnutritive, nonfood substances. Rumination disorder refers to the recurrent regurgitation of food, which can be seen in infants as well as throughout the life cycle. Pica and rumination disorder can be diagnosed with comorbid psychiatric conditions such as autism spectrum disorder, intellectual disability, and schizophrenia, as long as the eating disorder reaches a threshold of clinical significance.

Notably, DSM-5 clarifies a hierarchy of diagnoses so that only a single feeding or eating disorder diagnosis can be made for any particular individual (with the exception that pica can be comorbid with any other feeding or eating disorder). The overall eating disorder hierarchy is AN, BN, ARFID, BED, and rumination disorder. In other words, AN takes precedence over the others, and if AN is diagnosed, the individual cannot also have, for example, BED.

Suggested Readings

Stice E, Marti CN, Rohde P: Prevalence, incidence, impairment, and course of the proposed DSM-5 eating disorder diagnoses in an 8-year prospective community study of young women. J Abnorm Psychol 122(2):445–457, 2013 PubMed ID: 23148784

Striegel-Moore RH, Wonderlich SA, Walsh BT, Mitchell JE (eds): Developing an Evidence-Based Classification of Eating Disorders: Scientific Findings for DSM-5. Arlington, VA, American Psychiatric Association, 2011

Walsh BT: The enigmatic persistence of anorexia nervosa. Am J Psychiatry 170(5):477–484, 2013 PubMed ID: 23429750

Case 1: Stomachache

Susan Samuels, M.D.

Thomas, an 8-year-old boy with a mild to moderate intellectual disability, was brought into the emergency room (ER) by his parents after his abdominal pain of the past several weeks had worsened over the prior 24 hours. His parents reported that he had developed constipation, with only one bowel movement in the past week, and that he had vomited earlier in the day. Teachers at his special education classroom for children with intellectual disabilities had written a report earlier in the week indicating that Thomas had been having difficulties since soon after transferring from a similar school in Florida about 4 months earlier. The teachers and parents agreed that Thomas often looked distressed, rocking, crying, and clutching his stomach.

One week earlier, a pediatrician had diagnosed an acute exacerbation of chronic constipation. Use of a recommended over-the-counter laxative did not help, and Thomas began to complain of nighttime pain. The discomfort led to a diminished interest in his favorite hobbies, which were video games and sports. Instead, he tended to stay in his room, playing with army men figurines that he had inherited from his grandfather's collection. Aside from episodes of irritability and tearfulness, he was generally doing well in school, both in the classroom and on the playground. When not complaining of stomachaches, Thomas ate well and maintained his position at about the 40th percentile for height and weight on the growth curve.

Thomas's past medical history was significant for constipation and stomachaches, as well as intermittent headaches. All of these symptoms had worsened several months earlier, after the family moved from a house in semirural Florida into an old walk-up apartment in a large urban city. He shared a room with his younger brother (age 6 years), the product of a normal, unexpected pregnancy, who was enrolled in a regular education class at the local public school. Thomas said his brother was his "best friend." Thomas was adopted at birth, and nothing was known of his biological parents except that they were teenagers unable to care for the child.

On medical examination in the ER, Thomas was a well-groomed boy sitting on his mother's lap. He was crying and irritable and refused to speak to the examiner. Instead, he would repeat to his parents that his stomach hurt. On physical examination, he was afebrile and had stable vital signs. His physical examination was remarkable only for general abdominal tenderness, although he was difficult to assess because he cried uncontrollably through most of the exam.

An abdominal X ray revealed multiple small metallic particles throughout the gastrointestinal tract, initially suspected to be ingested high-lead paint flakes, as well as three 2-centimeter-long metallic objects in his stomach. A blood lead level was 20 µg/dL (whereas normal level for children is <5 µg/dL). More specific questioning revealed that Thomas, being constipated, often spent long stretches on the toilet by himself. His parents added that although the bathroom was in the process of being renovated, its paint was old and peeling. Consultants decided that the larger foreign bodies in the stomach might not safely pass and could be accounting for the constipation. Endoscopy successfully extricated three antique toy soldiers from Thomas's stomach.

Diagnoses

- Pica
- Intellectual disability, mild to moderate

Discussion

Thomas is an 8-year-old child with intellectual disability who was brought to an ER with abdominal pain, chronic constipation, irritability, and changes in mood and functioning. All of these symptoms followed his move to a new city and school 4 months earlier. The differential diagnosis for such complaints is broad and includes psychiatric causes, but the first priority is to do a thorough medical workup to search for sources of pain that the child might not be able to explain (e.g., ear infections, urinary tract infections).

When abdominal pain and constipation are the chief complaints, an abdominal radiograph generally reveals intestines full of stool. Such a result would prompt a more aggressive bowel regimen, as was recommended the week before by his pediatrician. Thomas's X ray, however, was unusual in that it revealed not only the residue of lead-based paint chips but also three small toy soldiers.

The persistent eating of nonnutritive, nonfood substances is the core feature of pica. To meet DSM-5 criteria, the ingestion must be severe enough to warrant clinical attention. Pica is most commonly comorbid with intellectual disability and autism spectrum disorder, although it can also be found in other disorders, such as schizophrenia and obsessive-compulsive disorder. As seen in Thomas, there is typically no aversion to food in general, and he continued to maintain his position on the growth chart.

Pica does not refer simply to the mouthing and occasional ingestion of nonfood objects that is common in infants, toddlers, and individuals with developmental delay. Instead, pica refers to chronic and clinically relevant ingestion of such inedible objects as clay, dirt, string, or cigarette butts. Pica can be extremely dangerous. In Thomas's case, for example, he could have suffered a gastrointestinal perforation from the soldiers. In addition, he was eating lead-based paint as well as the soldiers (which, being his grandfather's, could also have been made of lead). The acute lead exposure likely contributed to his abdominal pain, whereas chronic ingestion could be neurologically catastrophic in this boy who already has intellectual disability.

In addition to having the abdominal pain, Thomas was isolating himself from his classmates and brother and was irritable and tearful. It is possible that these are reflections of his pain, but they appear to be signs of psychological stress. The pica itself could also be a sign of stress, especially if it began only after the move from Florida. Psychosocial stressors frequently cause multiple physical symptoms in children, especially in those with intellectual disability. Thomas might also qualify, therefore, for a diagnosis of adjustment disorder with depressed mood. If his mood changes are determined to be secondary to the toxic levels of lead in his bloodstream, then a more accurate diagnosis might be a substance-induced depressive or anxiety disorder. In the ER setting, however, the clinician would likely defer making depressive, anxiety, or adjustment disorder diagnoses until having a chance to evaluate Thomas when he was not in acute abdominal distress.

Suggested Readings

Barrett RP: Atypical behavior: self-injury and pica, in Developmental-Behavioral Pediatrics: Evidence and Practice. Edited by Wolraich ML, Drotar DD, Dworkin PH, Perrin EC. Philadelphia, PA, Mosby-Elsevier, 2008, pp 871–886

Katz ER, DeMaso RR: Rumination, pica, and elimination (enuresis, encopresis) disorders, in Nelson Textbook of Pediatrics, 19th Edition. Edited by Kliegman RM, Stanton BF, St Geme J, et al. Philadelphia, PA, Elsevier/Saunders, 2011

Williams DE, McAdam D: Assessment, behavioral treatment, and prevention of pica: clinical guidelines and recommendations for practitioners. Res Dev Disabil 33(6):2050–2057, 2012 PubMed ID: 22750361

Case 2: Drifting Below the Growth Curve

Eve K. Freidl, M.D.
Evelyn Attia, M.D.

Uma, an 11-year-old girl in a gifted and talented school, was referred to an eating disorder specialist by a child psychiatrist who was concerned that Uma had drifted below the 10th percentile for weight. The psychiatrist had been treating Uma for perfectionistic traits that caused her significant anxiety. Their sessions focused on anxiety, not on eating behavior.

Uma's eating difficulties started at age 9, when she began refusing to eat and reporting a fear that she would vomit. At that time, her parents sought treatment from a pediatrician, who continued to evaluate her yearly, explaining that it was normal for children to go through phases. At age 9, Uma was above the 25th percentile for both height and weight (52 inches, 58 pounds), but by age 11, she had essentially stopped growing and had dropped to the 5th percentile on her growth curves (52.5 inches, 55 pounds).

The only child of two professional parents who had divorced 5 years earlier, Uma lived with her mother on weekdays and with her nearby father on weekends. Her medical history was significant for her premature birth at 34 weeks' gestation. She was slow to achieve her initial milestones but by age 2 was developmentally normal. Yearly physical examinations had been unremarkable with the exception of the recent decline of her growth trajectory. Uma had always been petite, but her height and weight had never fallen below the 25th percentile for stature and weight for age on the growth chart. Uma was a talented student who was well liked by her teachers. She had never had more than a few friends, but recently she had stopped socializing entirely and had been coming directly home after school, reporting that her stomach felt calmer when she was in her own home.

For the prior 2 years, Uma had eaten only very small amounts of food over very long durations of time. Her parents had tried to pique her interest by experimenting with foods from different cultures and of different colors and textures. None of this seemed effective in improving her appetite. They also tried to let her pick restaurants to try, but Uma had gradually refused to eat outside of either parent's home. Both parents reported a similar mealtime pattern: Uma would agree to sit at the table but then spent her time rearranging food on her plate, cutting food items into small pieces, and crying if urged to eat another bite.

When asked more about her fear of vomiting, Uma remembered one incident, at age 4, when she ate soup and her stomach became upset and then she subsequently vomited. More recently, Uma had developed fear of eating in public and ate no food during the school day. She denied any concerns about her appearance and only became aware of her low weight after her most recent visit to the pediatrician. When educated about the dangers of low body weight, Uma became tearful and expressed a clear desire to gain weight.

Diagnosis

• Avoidant/restrictive food intake disorder

Discussion

Uma is an 11-year-old girl who presents with a refusal to eat enough food to maintain her position on the growth curve. She fears vomiting, will not eat in public, and has gradually isolated herself from her friends. In contrast to individuals with anorexia nervosa (AN), Uma does not report any fear of gaining weight or becoming fat and does not deny the seriousness of her current low body weight. Her diagnosis, therefore, is avoidant/restrictive food intake disorder (ARFID), a new diagnosis in DSM-5. ARFID is a relatively broad category intended to describe a cluster of people who do not meet criteria for AN but whose avoidance or restriction of food leads to health problems, psychosocial dysfunction, and/or significant weight loss. In the case of children like Uma, the diminished food intake might result in a flattening of the growth trajectory rather than weight loss.

People with AN have a fear of gaining weight or of becoming fat, whereas people with ARFID lack a disturbance in body image. The distinction between ARFID and AN may be uncertain when individuals deny a fear of weight gain but instead offer diverse explanations for food restriction, such as somatic complaints (e.g., abdominal discomfort, fullness, lack of appetite), religious motives, desire for control, or desire for familial impact. Longitudinal assessment may be necessary to clarify the diagnosis, and ARFID may precede AN in some people.

A diagnosis of ARFID is likely to be applied primarily to children and adolescents, but people of any age can have this disorder. Three main subtypes have been described: inadequate overall intake in the presence of an emotional disturbance such that the emotional problem interferes with appetite and eating but the avoidance does not stem from a specific motive; restricted range of food intake (sometimes referred to as "picky eating"); and food avoidance due to a specific fear such as fear of swallowing (functional dysphagia), fear of poisoning, or fear of vomiting.

Uma fears going out and appears to avoid friends and social experiences. Such behavior might be consistent with a specific phobia, in that Uma specifically feared vomiting in public. Although specific phobia may be concurrent with an eating disorder, a diagnosis of ARFID is likely a more parsimonious explanation. As outlined in DSM-5, ARFID should be diagnosed in the presence of symptoms compatible with another diagnosis when the severity of the eating disturbance exceeds that routinely associated with the other condition and warrants additional clinical attention.

In Uma's case, a variety of other disorders should also be considered during the evaluation. These include medical, structural, and neurological disorders that can impede eating; obsessive-compulsive disorder; and depressive and anxiety disorders that might have emerged in the context of her parents' divorce and her progression toward puberty. Although any of these might be further explored, none of them seem immediately pertinent to Uma's weight loss.

Suggested Readings

Bryant-Waugh R, Markham L, Kreipe RE, et al: Feeding and eating disorders in childhood. Int J Eat Disord 43(2):98–111, 2010 PubMed ID: 20063374

Kreipe RE, Palomaki A: Beyond picky eating: avoidant/restrictive food intake disorder. Curr Psychiatry Rep 14(4):421–431, 2012 PubMed ID: 22665043

Case 3: Headaches and Fatigue

Jennifer J. Thomas, Ph.D.
Anne E. Becker, M.D., Ph.D.

Valerie Gaspard was a 20-year-old single black woman who had recently immigrated to the United States from West Africa with her family to do missionary work. She presented to her primary care physician complaining of frequent headaches and chronic fatigue. Her physical examination was unremarkable except that her weight was only 78 pounds and her height was 5 feet 1 inch, resulting in a body mass index (BMI) of 14.7 kg/m^2, and she had missed her last menstrual period. Unable to find a medical explanation for Ms. Gaspard's symptoms, and feeling concerned about her extremely low weight, the physician referred Ms. Gaspard to the hospital eating disorders program.

Upon presentation for psychiatric evaluation, Ms. Gaspard was cooperative and pleasant. She expressed concern about her low weight and denied fear of weight gain or body image disturbance: "I know I need to gain weight. I'm too skinny," she said. Ms. Gaspard reported that she had weighed 97 pounds prior to moving to the United States and said she felt "embarrassed" when her family members and even strangers told her she had grown too thin. Notably, everyone else in her U.S.-dwelling extended family was either of normal weight or overweight.

Despite her apparent motivation to correct her malnutrition, Ms. Gaspard's dietary recall revealed that she was consuming only 600 calories per day. The day before the evaluation, for example, she had eaten only a small bowl of macaroni pasta, a plate of steamed broccoli, and a cup of black beans. Her fluid intake was also quite limited, typically consisting of only two or three glasses of water daily.

Ms. Gaspard provided multiple reasons for her poor intake. The first was lack of appetite: "My brain doesn't even signal that I'm hungry," she said. "I have no desire to eat throughout the whole day." The second was postprandial bloating and nausea:

"I just feel so uncomfortable after eating." The third was the limited choice of foods permitted by her religion, which advocates a vegetarian diet. "My body is not really my own. It is a temple of God," she explained. The fourth reason was that her preferred sources of vegetarian protein (e.g., tofu, processed meat substitutes) were not affordable within her meager budget. Ms. Gaspard had not completed high school and made very little money working at a secretarial job at her church.

Ms. Gaspard denied any other symptoms of disordered eating, including binge eating, purging, or other behaviors intended to promote weight loss. However, with regard to exercise, she reported that she walked for approximately 3–4 hours per day. She denied that her activity was motivated by a desire to burn calories. Instead, Ms. Gaspard stated that because she did not have a car and disliked waiting for the bus, she traveled on foot to all work and leisure activities.

Ms. Gaspard reported no other notable psychiatric symptoms apart from her inadequate food intake and excessive physical activity. She appeared euthymic and did not report any symptoms of depression. She denied using alcohol or illicit drugs. She noted that her concentration was poor but expressed hope that a herbal supplement she had just begun taking would improve her memory. When queried about past treatment history, she reported that she had briefly seen a dietitian about a year earlier when her family began "nagging" her about her low weight, but she had not viewed the meetings as helpful.

Diagnosis

• Anorexia nervosa, restricting type

Discussion

Ms. Gaspard's most appropriate DSM-5 diagnosis is anorexia nervosa (AN). Although her history suggests alternative explanations for her cachectic presentation, none is as compelling as AN. For example, avoidant/restrictive food intake disorder, newly named with revised criteria in DSM-5, could also present with an eating disturbance, significant malnutrition, and either a lack of interest in or an aversion to eating triggered by or associated with a range of physical complaints, including gastrointestinal discomfort. However, Ms. Gaspard's bloating and nausea are a red herring: both are common in AN, where they can be idiopathic or associated with delayed gastric emptying or whole-gut transit time. Similarly, although major depressive disorder can also be associated with appetite loss, Ms. Gaspard is euthymic and actively engaged in her missionary work. Lastly, although Ms. Gaspard's limited access to food and transportation may contribute to her malnutrition and excessive physical activity, it is notable that no one else in her family (with whom she shares communal resources) is underweight.

Because Ms. Gaspard does not engage in binge eating (i.e., she denies eating large amounts of food while feeling out of control) or purging (i.e., she denies self-induced vomiting or abuse of enemas, laxatives, diuretics, or other medications), her presentation is consistent with the restricting subtype of AN. An elevated risk for an eating disorder following immigration from a culturally non-Western to a Western country has been described for some populations, attributed to increased exposure to Western beauty ideals as well as stressors associated with acculturation. Although Ms. Gaspard would not have met DSM-IV criteria for AN because of her lack of fat phobia and her continued (albeit irregular) menses, she meets revised DSM-5 criteria for AN.

The first criterion for AN is significantly low weight. Ms. Gaspard's BMI of 14.7 places her below the first BMI centile for U.S. females of her age and height. Furthermore, her BMI is well below the World Health Organization's lower limit of 18.5 kg/m^2 for adults. Her weight is so low that her menses have become irregular. It is important to note that amenorrhea (i.e., lack of menses for 3 months or more) was a DSM-IV criterion for AN but was omitted from DSM-5 due to research suggesting that low-weight eating-disorder patients who menstruate regularly exhibit psychopathology commensurate with that of their counterparts with amenorrhea.

A second criterion for AN is either an intense fear of fatness or persistent behavior that interferes with weight gain despite a significantly low weight. Ms. Gaspard's rationales for food refusal are inconsistent with the intense fear of weight gain that DSM-IV previously characterized as the sine qua non of AN. However, many low-weight patients—especially those from culturally non-Western backgrounds—do not explicitly endorse weight and shape concerns.

Culture-based differences—including prevailing local norms that govern many factors, including dietary and meal patterns, aesthetic ideals for body shape and weight, embodiment of core cultural symbols and social relations, self-agency and self-presentation, and somatic idioms of distress—potentially influence the experience, manifestation, and articulation of eating pathology. For example, a clinical narrative that links restrictive eating behaviors to weight management goals can be easily formulated for a patient whose social context associates prestige with thinness, stigmatizes obesity, and assigns high value to achievement and autonomy.

The determinative cultural underpinnings of conventional AN presentation are perhaps best illustrated in Sing Lee's work from Hong Kong documenting "non-fat-phobic anorexia nervosa," a variant of eating disorder that strongly resembles DSM-IV AN except for its absent fear of weight gain. Lee and colleagues argued that fear of fatness had insufficient cultural salience for many of their patients, who rationalized extreme dietary restriction differently but nonetheless reached a dangerously low weight. Evidence that the absence of fat phobia may be associated with a more benign clinical course raises compelling questions about not just cultural mediation, but also cultural moderation of eating pathology. Globalized commerce and communication have opened avenues for broad exposure to what Sing Lee termed a "culture of modernity," and eating disorders are now recognized as having wide geographical distribution. The amendment in DSM-5 of AN Criterion B now encompasses individuals like Ms. Gaspard who exhibit persistent behavior that interferes with weight gain, even if they do not explicitly endorse fat phobia.

Indeed, Ms. Gaspard's low food intake (600 calories per day) and high level of physical activity (3–4 hours per day) are clearly at odds with her stated desire to gain weight, however earnest her pronouncements may sound. Moreover, her myriad rationales for her restricted dietary intake (ranging from lack of hunger to forgetfulness to lack of resources) slightly undermine the credibility of each individual one. Following Ms. Gaspard over time to ascertain that her behaviors are persistent would help confirm the AN diagnosis, but her clinical history suggests that when Ms. Gaspard has previously been confronted about her low weight (i.e., by her family, by the dietitian), she has been either unwilling or unable to implement changes that would restore her to a healthy weight.

A diagnosis of AN also requires that a third criterion be met: a disturbance in the experience of one's body or shape, undue influence of that weight or shape on self-evaluation, and/or a lack of recognition of the seriousness of low weight. Ms. Gaspard denies an altered self-image and says she is worried about her low weight. However, her lack of follow-through with an earlier dietary intervention and her subsequent presentation to primary care to manage the symptoms of her dehydration and malnutrition (i.e., headaches, fatigue, poor concentration) suggest that she may not grasp the seriousness of her low weight. Furthermore, Ms. Gaspard's characterization of her family's appropriate concern as "nagging" supports that she does not recognize the health impacts of her significantly low weight.

Suggested Readings

Becker AE, Thomas JJ, Pike KM: Should non-fat-phobic anorexia nervosa be included in DSM-V? Int J Eat Disord 42(7):620–635, 2009 PubMed ID: 19655370

Benini L, Todesco T, Dalle Grave R, et al: Gastric emptying in patients with restricting and binge/purging subtypes of anorexia nervosa. Am J Gastroenterol 99(8):1448–1454, 2004 PubMed ID: 15307858

Centers for Disease Control and Prevention, National Center for Health Statistics: CDC growth charts: United States. Advance Data No. 314. Vital and Health Statistics of the Centers for Disease Control and Prevention. May 30, 2000. Available at: http://www.cdc.gov/growthcharts/data/set1clinical/cj41c024.pdf. Accessed May 6, 2013.

Lee S: Self-starvation in context: towards a culturally sensitive understanding of anorexia nervosa. Soc Sci Med 41(1):25–36, 1995 PubMed ID: 7667670

Lee S: Reconsidering the status of anorexia nervosa as a Western culture–bound syndrome. Soc Sci Med 42(1):21–34, 1996 PubMed ID: 8745105

Roberto CA, Steinglass J, Mayer LE, et al: The clinical significance of amenorrhea as a diagnostic criterion for anorexia nervosa. Int J Eat Disord 41(6):559–563, 2008 PubMed ID: 18454485

van Hoeken D, Veling W, Smink FR, et al: The incidence of anorexia nervosa in Netherlands Antilles immigrants in the Netherlands. Eur Eat Disord Rev 18(5):399–403, 2010 PubMed ID: 20821741

Case 4: Vomiting

James E. Mitchell, M.D.

Wanda Hoffman was a 24-year-old white woman who presented with a chief complaint: "I have problems throwing up." These symptoms had their roots in early adolescence, when she began dieting despite a normal body mass index (BMI). At age 18 she went away to college and began to overeat in the context of new academic and social demands. A 10-pound weight gain led her to routinely skip breakfast. She often skipped lunch as well, but then—famished—would overeat in the late afternoon and evening.

The overeating episodes intensified, in both frequency and volume of food, and Ms. Hoffman increasingly felt out of control. Worried that the binges would lead to weight gain, she started inducing vomiting, a practice she learned about in a magazine. She first thought this pattern of behavior to be quite acceptable and saw self-induced vomiting as a way of controlling her fears about weight gain. The pattern became entrenched: morning food restriction followed by binge eating followed by self-induced vomiting.

Ms. Hoffman continued to function adequately in college and to maintain friendships, always keeping her behavior a secret from those around her. After college graduation, she returned to her hometown and took a job at a local bank. Despite renewing old friendships and dating and enjoying her work, she often did not feel well. She described diminished energy and poor sleep, as well as various abdominal complaints, including, at different times, constipation and diarrhea. She frequently made excuses to avoid friends, and she became progressively more socially isolated. Her mood deteriorated, and she found herself feeling worthless. At times, she wished she were dead. She decided to break out of this downward spiral by getting a psychiatric referral from her internist.

On mental status examination, the patient was a well-developed, well-nourished female, in no apparent distress. Her BMI was normal at 23. She was coherent, cooperative, and goal directed. She often felt sad and worried but denied feeling depressed. She denied an intention to kill herself but did sometimes think life was not worth living. She denied confusion. Her cognition was intact, and her insight and judgment were considered fair.

Diagnoses

- Bulimia nervosa
- Major depressive disorder

Discussion

Ms. Hoffman presents a fairly classic history for bulimia nervosa (BN). Like 90% of patients with BN, Ms. Hoffman is female, and, as is usual, her symptoms began when she was in her late teens or early 20s. One reason for this age at onset is the stress of entering college or the workforce. Genetics and environment also play a role, but it is not entirely clear why certain young people develop BN while others do not, despite equivalent amounts of body dissatisfaction.

The hallmark of the illness is binge eating, which is usually defined as eating an inappropriately large amount of food in a discrete period of time (e.g., at a meal), in conjunction with a sense of loss of control while eating. Although food portions are typically large in BN, the predominant feature for many people is the sense of loss of control.

Along with the binge eating, the vast majority of patients engage in self-induced vomiting. This behavior usually begins out of fear that the binge eating will result in weight gain, with the subsequent vomiting seen as a way of eliminating this risk. Early in the course of the illness, most patients induce vomiting with their fingers, but they often develop the capacity to vomit at will. Some patients with BN may also use laxatives to induce diarrhea; this method may induce a sense of weight loss, but laxatives are actually more effective at inducing dehydration, with its accompanying physical symptoms and medical risk. Some individuals with BN also use diuretics, and many experiment with diet pills.

Most people with BN tend to seek help because of complications of the disorder rather than dissatisfaction with the eating behavior. For example, medical complications commonly include dehydration and electrolyte abnormalities, particularly hypochloremia and metabolic alkalosis, and, more rarely, hypokalemia. These complications can lead to feelings of fatigue, headache, and poor concentration. Rare but serious medical complications include gastric dilatation and esophageal rupture.

In addition to the eating disorder, Ms. Hoffman presents with depressed mood, anhedonia, poor sleep, low energy, physical complaints, feelings of worthlessness, and diminished concentration. She denies suicidal intent or plan, but she does have thoughts of death. She meets criteria, therefore, for a DSM-5 major depressive disorder. Depression is commonly comorbid with BN. Other common comorbidities include anxiety disorders, substance use problems (often involving alcohol, and personality disorders).

Although Ms. Hoffman sought help from a psychiatrist, she did so through her internist, and it is common for people with BN to present to their primary care physicians with vague medical complaints. Interestingly, the health practitioners who are often in the best position to identify patients with BN are dentists, who find evidence of obvious enamel erosion.

Suggested Readings

Peat C, Mitchell JE, Hoek HW, et al: Validity and utility of subtyping anorexia nervosa. Int J Eat Disord 42(7):590–594, 2009 PubMed ID: 19598270
van Hoeken D, Veling W, Sinke S, et al: The validity and utility of subtyping bulimia nervosa. Int J Eat Disord 42(7):595–602, 2009 PubMed ID: 19621467
Wonderlich SA, Gordon KH, Mitchell JE, et al: The validity and clinical utility of binge eating disorder. Int J Eat Disord 42(8):687–705, 2009 PubMed ID: 19621466

Case 5: Weight Gain

Susan L. McElroy, M.D.

Yasmine Isherwood, a 55-year-old married woman, had been in psychiatric treatment for 6 months for an episode of major depression. She had responded well to a combination of psychotherapy and medications (fluoxetine and bupropion), but she began to complain of weight gain. She was at her "highest weight ever," which was 140 pounds (her height was 5 feet 5 inches, so her BMI was 23.3).

The psychiatrist embarked on a clarification of Ms. Isherwood's eating history, which was marked by recurrent, distressing episodes of uncontrollable eating of large amounts of food. The overeating was not new but seemed to have worsened while she was taking antidepressants. She reported that the episodes occurred two or three times per week, usually between the time she arrived home from work and the time her husband did so. These "eating jags" were notable for a sense that she was out of control. She ate rapidly and alone, until uncomfortably full. She would then feel depressed, tired, and disgusted with herself. She usually binged on healthy food but also had "sugar binges" where she ate primarily sweets, especially ice cream and candy. She denied current or past self-induced vomiting, fasting, or misuse of laxatives, diuretics, or weight-loss agents. She reported exercising for an hour almost every day but denied being "addicted" to it. She did report that in her late 20s, she had become a competitive runner. At that time, she had often run 10-kilometer races and averaged about 35 miles per week, despite a lingering foot injury that eventually forced her to shift to swimming, biking, and the elliptical machine.

Ms. Isherwood stated that she had binged on food "for as long as I can remember." She was "chunky" as a child but stayed at a normal weight throughout high school (120–125 pounds) because she was so active. She denied a history of anorexia nervosa. At age 28, she reached her lowest adult weight of 113 pounds. At that point, she felt "vital, healthy, and in control."

In her mid-30s, she had a major depressive episode that lasted 2 years. She had a severely depressed mood, did not talk, "closed down," stayed in bed, was very fatigued, slept more than usual, and was unable to function. This was one of the few times in her life that the binge eating stopped and she lost weight. She denied a history of hypomanic or manic episodes. Although she lived with frequent sadness, she denied other serious depressive episodes until the past year. She denied a history of suicidal ideation, suicide attempts, and any significant use of alcohol, tobacco, or illicit substances.

The evaluation revealed a well-nourished, well-developed female who was coherent and cooperative. Her speech was fluent and not pressured. She had a mildly depressed mood but had a reactive affect with appropriate smiles. She denied guilt, suicidality, and hopelessness. She said her energy was normal except for post-binge fatigue. She denied psychosis and confusion. Her cognition was normal. Her medical history was unremarkable, and physical examination and basic laboratory test results provided by her internist were within normal limits.

Diagnoses

- Binge-eating disorder, mild
- Major depressive disorder, recurrent, in remission

Discussion

Ms. Isherwood describes overeating episodes that are marked by a sense of being out of control. She eats rapidly and until overly full. She eats alone and feels disgusted and distressed afterward. These episodes occur several times per week and do not involve inappropriate compensatory behaviors such as vomiting or use of laxatives. She conforms, therefore, to the new DSM-5 definition of binge-eating disorder (BED).

Although BED shares features with bulimia nervosa (BN) and obesity, it is distinguishable from both conditions. Compared to obese individuals without binge eating, obese individuals with BED have greater weight concerns and higher rates of mood, anxiety, and substance use disorders. Compared to individuals with BN, individuals with BED have lower weight concerns, greater rates of obesity, and lower rates of associated mood, anxiety, and substance use disorders. DSM-5 criteria for BED have been broadened from the provisional DSM-IV criteria. Instead of a requirement of two binge episodes per week for 6 months, DSM-5 requires one episode per week for 3 months. This shift represents an example of the sort of research that examines symptomatic clustering. In this case, it became apparent that individuals with less frequent and less persistent binge episodes were quite similar to people with slightly more frequent and more persistent episodes. Ms. Isherwood reports two or three episodes per week, which would put her in the mild category.

Although a diagnosis of BED should not be given in the presence of either BN or AN, patients with BED can have past histories of other eating disorders as well as infrequent inappropriate compensatory behaviors. For example, Ms. Isherwood recalled a period of time in her 20s when she was running frequent races and running 35 miles per week with a chronic foot ailment. Even though she recalls feeling "vital, healthy, and in control" during that period of time, she may also have had BN if that period included both binge eating and competitive running that was intended to compensate for the bingeing.

BED patients often seek treatment initially for obesity (BMI≥30), but clinical samples indicate that up to one-third of patients with BED are not obese. Non-obese patients with BED are more similar to than different from their obese counterparts, although they are more likely to engage in both healthy and unhealthy weight loss behaviors. It is possible that Ms. Isherwood maintained a normal weight despite her extensive binge-eating history because of her regular exercise regimen. It is also possible that Ms. Isherwood's excessive running was spurred by an episode of hypomania; about 15% of patients with bipolar II disorder have an eating disorder, and BED is the most common.

BED is often associated with mood, anxiety, substance use, and impulse-control disorders. Although Ms. Isherwood denies any history of alcohol or drug misuse, she has a history of recurrent major depressive disorder. Although the case does not go into detail, it would be useful to explore the connection between Ms. Isherwood's eating habits and her depressive symptoms. Major depression itself can lead to excess eating, but if both BED and depression are present, both should be diagnosed. Finally, the history does not discuss personality, but bingeing is included in the impulse-control criterion for borderline personality disorder. If full criteria for both are met, then both should be diagnosed.

Suggested Readings

Goldschmidt AB, Le Grange D, Powers P, et al: Eating disorder symptomatology in normal-weight vs. obese individuals with binge eating disorder. Obesity (Silver Spring) 19(7):1515–1518, 2011 PubMed ID: 21331066

Hudson JI, Hiripi E, Pope HG Jr, et al: The prevalence and correlates of eating disorders in the National Comorbidity Survey Replication. Biol Psychiatry 61(3):348–358, 2007 PubMed ID: 16815322

Wonderlich SA, Gordon KH, Mitchell JE, et al: The validity and clinical utility of binge eating disorder. Int J Eat Disord 42(8):687–705, 2009 PubMed ID: 19621466

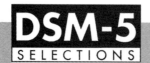

Feeding and Eating Disorders

DSM-5® Self-Exam Questions

1. Which DSM-5 diagnosis replaced the DSM-IV diagnosis of feeding disorder of infancy or early childhood?

   A. Anorexia nervosa.
   B. Unspecified feeding or eating disorder.
   C. Anorexia nervosa of early childhood.
   D. Avoidant/restrictive food intake disorder.
   E. Pica.

2. Which of the following statements about DSM-5 changes in the diagnostic criteria for anorexia nervosa is *true?*

   A. The requirement for menorrhagia has been eliminated.
   B. The requirement for amenorrhea has been eliminated.
   C. The requirements for amenorrhea and menorrhagia have been eliminated.
   D. Low body weight is no longer required.
   E. Developmental stage is no longer a significant issue.

3. Which of the following statements about DSM-5 changes in the diagnostic criteria for bulimia nervosa is *true?*

   A. There is an increase in the required numbers of binge-eating episodes and inappropriate compensatory behaviors per week, from twice to three times weekly.
   B. There is an increase in the numbers of episodes of using ipecac or vomiting per week, from three to four.
   C. There is a reduction in the required minimum frequency of binge eating and inappropriate compensatory behavior frequency, from twice to once weekly.
   D. There is a requirement for an episode of pica, at least once in the last year.
   E. There is a requirement for electrolyte imbalances to be demonstrated at least twice in the past 2 years.

4. What is the minimum average frequency of binge eating required for a diagnosis of DSM-5 binge-eating disorder?

   A. Once weekly for the last 3 months.
   B. Once weekly for the last 4 months.

    C. Every other week for the last 3 months.

    D. Every other week for the last 4 months.

    E. Once a month for the last 3 months.

5. In avoidant/restrictive food intake disorder, the eating or feeding disturbance is manifested by persistent failure to meet appropriate nutritional and/or energy needs associated with one or more of four specified features. Which of the following options correctly lists these four features?

    A. Manic or hypomanic symptoms; ruminative behaviors; compulsive thoughts; marked interference with psychosocial functioning.

    B. Significant weight loss; significant nutritional deficiency; dependence on enteral feeding or oral nutritional supplements; marked interference with psychosocial functioning.

    C. Significant weight loss; ruminative behaviors; delusions or hallucinations; manic or hypomanic symptoms.

    D. Significant nutritional deficiency; increased use of alcohol or other substances; manic or hypomanic symptoms; delusions or hallucinations.

    E. Dependence on enteral feeding or oral nutritional supplements; ruminative behaviors; delusions or hallucinations; manic or hypomanic symptoms.

6. Which of the following statements about onset and prevalence of avoidant/restrictive food intake disorder is *true*?

    A. The disorder occurs mostly in females, with onset typically in older adolescence.

    B. The disorder occurs mostly in males, with onset typically in early childhood.

    C. The disorder is more common in childhood and more common in females than in males.

    D. The disorder is more common in childhood and equally common in males and females.

    E. The disorder is extremely common in elderly adults, who often manifest an age-related reduction in intake.

7. A 45-year-old woman had a choking episode 3 years ago after eating salad. Since that time she has been afraid to eat a wide range of foods, fearing that she will choke. This fear has affected her functionality and her ability to eat out with friends and has contributed to weight loss. Which diagnosis best fits this clinical picture?

    A. Bulimia nervosa.

    B. Schizophrenia.

    C. Avoidant/restrictive food intake disorder.

    D. Binge-eating disorder.

    E. Adjustment disorder.

8. What are the two subtypes of anorexia nervosa?

    A. Restricting type and binge-eating/purging type.
    B. Energy-sparing type and binge-eating/purging type.
    C. Low-calorie/low-carbohydrate type and restricting type.
    D. Low-carbohydrate/low-fat type and restricting type.
    E. Restricting type and low-weight type.

9. What are the three essential diagnostic features of anorexia nervosa?

    A. Persistently low self-confidence, intense fear of becoming fat, and disturbance in motivation.
    B. Low self-esteem, disturbance in self-perceived weight or shape, and persistent energy restriction.
    C. Restricted affect, disturbance in motivation, and low calorie intake.
    D. Persistent restriction of energy intake, intense fear of becoming fat, and disturbance in self-perceived weight or shape.
    E. Persistent lack of weight gain, disturbance in motivation, and restricted affect.

10. What laboratory abnormalities are commonly found in individuals with anorexia nervosa?

    A. Elevated blood urea nitrogen (BUN); low triiodothyronine (T_3); hyperadrenocorticism; low serum estrogen (females) or testosterone (males); bradycardia; low bone mineral density.
    B. Low BUN; hypercholesterolemia; high thyroxine (T_4); hypoadrenocorticism; short QTc; low bone mineral density.
    C. Blast cells; thrombocytosis; hyperphosphatemia; hypoamylasemia; high serum estrogen (females) or testosterone (males).
    D. Hyperzincemia; hypermagnesemia; hyperchloremia; hyperkalemia.
    E. C and D.

11. A 27-year-old graduate student has a 10-year history of anorexia nervosa. Her boyfriend is quite concerned because she has extreme fears related to cleanliness. She washes her hands more than 12 times a day and is excessively worried about contamination. What would be the best decision by the mental health professional at this point regarding these symptoms?

    A. Assume that the patient's obsessive-compulsive symptoms are related to her anorexia nervosa.
    B. Further evaluate the obsessive-compulsive features, because if they are not related to anorexia nervosa, a new diagnosis of obsessive-compulsive disorder might be warranted.
    C. Ask the patient to wait 1 year and see how this evolves.
    D. Make a diagnosis of body dysmorphic disorder.
    E. Refer the patient for a colonoscopy.

12. What are the three essential diagnostic features of bulimia nervosa?

    A. Recurrent episodes of binge eating; recurrent inappropriate compensatory behaviors to prevent weight gain; self-evaluation that is unduly influenced by body shape and weight.

    B. Recurrent restriction of food; self-evaluation that is unduly influenced by body shape and weight; mood instability.

    C. Delusions regarding body habitus; obsessional focus on food; recurrent purging.

    D. Hypomanic symptoms for 1 month; mood instability; self-evaluation that is unduly influenced by body shape and weight.

    E. Self-evaluation that is unduly influenced by body shape and weight; history of anorexia nervosa; recurrent inappropriate compensatory behaviors to gain weight.

13. What are the subtypes of bulimia nervosa?

    A. Restrictive.

    B. Purging.

    C. Restrictive and purging.

    D. None.

    E. With normal weight/abnormal weight.

14. What minimum average frequency of binge eating is required to qualify for a diagnosis of binge-eating disorder?

    A. At least once a week for 3 months.

    B. At least twice a week for 3 months.

    C. At least once a week for 6 months.

    D. At least twice a week for 6 months.

    E. None of the above.

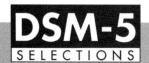

Feeding and Eating Disorders

DSM-5® Self-Exam Answer Guide

1. Which DSM-5 diagnosis replaced the DSM-IV diagnosis of feeding disorder of infancy or early childhood?

   A. Anorexia nervosa.
   B. Unspecified feeding or eating disorder.
   C. Anorexia nervosa of early childhood.
   D. Avoidant/restrictive food intake disorder.
   E. Pica.

   Correct Answer: D. Avoidant/restrictive food intake disorder.

   Explanation: Because of the elimination of the DSM-IV chapter "Disorders Usually First Diagnosed During Infancy, Childhood, or Adolescence," the DSM-5 Feeding and Eating Disorders chapter describes several disorders found in the DSM-IV section "Feeding and Eating Disorders of Infancy or Early Childhood," such as *pica* and *rumination disorder.* The DSM-IV category *feeding disorder of infancy or early childhood* has been renamed *avoidant/restrictive food intake disorder,* and the criteria are significantly expanded.

   1—Appendix / Highlights of Changes From DSM-IV to DSM-5 (p. 813)

2. Which of the following statements about DSM-5 changes in the diagnostic criteria for anorexia nervosa is *true?*

   A. The requirement for menorrhagia has been eliminated.
   B. The requirement for amenorrhea has been eliminated.
   C. The requirements for amenorrhea and menorrhagia have been eliminated.
   D. Low body weight is no longer required.
   E. Developmental stage is no longer a significant issue.

   Correct Answer: B. The requirement for amenorrhea has been eliminated.

   Explanation: The core diagnostic criteria for anorexia nervosa are conceptually unchanged from DSM-IV with one exception: the requirement for amenorrhea is eliminated. As in DSM-IV, individuals with this disorder are required by Criterion A to be at a significantly low body weight for their developmental stage.

The wording of the criterion is changed for clarification, and guidance regarding how to judge whether an individual is at or below a significantly low weight is provided in the text. In DSM-5, Criterion B is expanded to include not only overtly expressed fear of weight gain but also persistent behavior that interferes with weight gain.

2—Appendix / Highlights of Changes From DSM-IV to DSM-5 (p. 813)

3. Which of the following statements about DSM-5 changes in the diagnostic criteria for bulimia nervosa is *true?*

    A. There is an increase in the required numbers of binge-eating episodes and inappropriate compensatory behaviors per week, from twice to three times weekly.
    B. There is an increase in the numbers of episodes of using ipecac or vomiting per week, from three to four.
    C. There is a reduction in the required minimum frequency of binge eating and inappropriate compensatory behavior frequency, from twice to once weekly.
    D. There is a requirement for an episode of pica, at least once in the last year.
    E. There is a requirement for electrolyte imbalances to be demonstrated at least twice in the past 2 years.

Correct Answer: C. There is a reduction in the required minimum frequency of binge eating and inappropriate compensatory behavior frequency, from twice to once weekly.

Explanation: The only change in the DSM-IV criteria for bulimia nervosa is a reduction in the required minimum average frequency of binge eating and inappropriate compensatory behavior frequency from twice to once weekly.

3—Appendix / Highlights of Changes From DSM-IV to DSM-5 (p. 813)

4. What is the minimum average frequency of binge eating required for a diagnosis of DSM-5 binge-eating disorder?

    A. Once weekly for the last 3 months.
    B. Once weekly for the last 4 months.
    C. Every other week for the last 3 months.
    D. Every other week for the last 4 months.
    E. Once a month for the last 3 months.

Correct Answer: A. Once weekly for the last 3 months.

Explanation: Binge eating is reliably associated with obesity and overweight status in individuals who seek treatment. The extensive research that followed the promulgation of preliminary criteria for binge-eating disorder in Appendix B of DSM-IV documented the clinical utility and validity of binge-eating disorder. The only significant difference from the preliminary criteria is that the minimum average frequency of binge eating required for diagnosis is once weekly over the last 3 months, which is identical to the frequency criterion for bulimia nervosa (rather than at least 2 days a week for 6 months in DSM-IV).

4—Appendix / Highlights of Changes From DSM-IV to DSM-5 (p. 813)

5. In avoidant/restrictive food intake disorder, the eating or feeding disturbance is manifested by persistent failure to meet appropriate nutritional and/or energy needs associated with one or more of four specified features. Which of the following options correctly lists these four features?

   A. Manic or hypomanic symptoms; ruminative behaviors; compulsive thoughts; marked interference with psychosocial functioning.
   B. Significant weight loss; significant nutritional deficiency; dependence on enteral feeding or oral nutritional supplements; marked interference with psychosocial functioning.
   C. Significant weight loss; ruminative behaviors; delusions or hallucinations; manic or hypomanic symptoms.
   D. Significant nutritional deficiency; increased use of alcohol or other substances; manic or hypomanic symptoms; delusions or hallucinations.
   E. Dependence on enteral feeding or oral nutritional supplements; ruminative behaviors; delusions or hallucinations; manic or hypomanic symptoms.

Correct Answer: B. Significant weight loss; significant nutritional deficiency; dependence on enteral feeding or oral nutritional supplements; marked interference with psychosocial functioning.

Explanation: Avoidant/restrictive food intake disorder replaces and extends the DSM-IV diagnosis of feeding disorder of infancy or early childhood. The main diagnostic feature of avoidant/restrictive food intake disorder is avoidance or restriction of food intake (Criterion A) manifested by clinically significant failure to meet requirements for nutrition or insufficient energy intake through oral intake of food. One or more of the following key features must be present: significant weight loss, significant nutritional deficiency (or related health impact), dependence on enteral feeding or oral nutritional supplements, or marked interference with psychosocial functioning. The determination of whether weight loss is significant (Criterion A1) is a clinical judgment; instead of losing weight, children and adolescents who have not completed growth may not maintain weight or height increases along their developmental trajectory.

Determination of significant nutritional deficiency (Criterion A2) is also based on clinical assessment (e.g., assessment of dietary intake, physical examination, and laboratory testing). In severe cases, particularly in infants, malnutrition can be life threatening. "Dependence" on enteral feeding or oral nutritional supplements (Criterion A3) means that supplementary feeding is required to sustain adequate intake. Examples of individuals requiring supplementary feeding include infants with failure to thrive who require nasogastric tube feeding, children with neurodevelopmental disorders who are dependent on nutritionally complete supplements, and individuals who rely on gastrostomy tube feeding or complete oral nutrition supplements in the absence of an underlying medical condition.

5—Avoidant/Restrictive Food Intake Disorder / Diagnostic Features (pp. 334–335)

6. Which of the following statements about onset and prevalence of avoidant/ restrictive food intake disorder is *true?*

     A. The disorder occurs mostly in females, with onset typically in older adolescence.
     B. The disorder occurs mostly in males, with onset typically in early childhood.
     C. The disorder is more common in childhood and more common in females than in males.
     D. The disorder is more common in childhood and equally common in males and females.
     E. The disorder is extremely common in elderly adults, who often manifest an age-related reduction in intake.

Correct Answer: D. The disorder is more common in childhood and equally common in males and females.

Explanation: Avoidant/restrictive food intake disorder is equally common in males and females in infancy and early childhood. The disorder manifests more commonly in children than in adults, and there may be a long delay between onset and clinical presentation. Avoidant/restrictive food intake disorder does not include avoidance or restriction of food intake related to lack of availability of food or to cultural practices (e.g., religious fasting or normal dieting) (Criterion B), nor does it include developmentally normal behaviors (e.g., picky eating in toddlers, reduced intake in older adults).

6—Avoidant/Restrictive Food Intake Disorder / Diagnostic Features (pp. 334–335)

7. A 45-year-old woman had a choking episode 3 years ago after eating salad. Since that time she has been afraid to eat a wide range of foods, fearing that she will choke. This fear has affected her functionality and her ability to eat out with friends and has contributed to weight loss. Which diagnosis best fits this clinical picture?

     A. Bulimia nervosa.
     B. Schizophrenia.
     C. Avoidant/restrictive food intake disorder.
     D. Binge-eating disorder.
     E. Adjustment disorder.

Correct Answer: C. Avoidant/restrictive food intake disorder.

Explanation: Food avoidance or restriction may also represent a conditioned negative response associated with food intake following, or in anticipation of, an aversive experience, such as choking; a traumatic investigation, usually involving the gastrointestinal tract (e.g., esophagoscopy); or repeated vomiting. The terms *functional dysphagia* and *globus hystericus* have also been used for such conditions.

7—Avoidant/Restrictive Food Intake Disorder / Diagnostic Features (pp. 334–335)

8. What are the two subtypes of anorexia nervosa?

   A. Restricting type and binge-eating/purging type.
   B. Energy-sparing type and binge-eating/purging type.
   C. Low-calorie/low-carbohydrate type and restricting type.
   D. Low-carbohydrate/low-fat type and restricting type.
   E. Restricting type and low-weight type.

Correct Answer: A. Restricting type and binge-eating/purging type.

Explanation: The subtype specifiers describe the primary mode of weight loss used for the past 3 months. In the restricting subtype of anorexia nervosa, weight loss is accomplished primarily through dieting, fasting, and/or excessive exercise; in the binge-eating/purging subtype, it is accomplished through recurrent episodes of binge eating or purging behavior (i.e., self-induced vomiting or the misuse of laxatives, diuretics, or enemas).

   Most individuals with the binge-eating/purging type of anorexia nervosa who binge eat also purge through self-induced vomiting or the misuse of laxatives, diuretics, or enemas. Some individuals with this subtype of anorexia nervosa do not binge eat but do regularly purge after the consumption of small amounts of food. Crossover between the subtypes over the course of the disorder is not uncommon; therefore, subtype description should be used to describe current symptoms rather than longitudinal course.

8—Anorexia Nervosa / diagnostic criteria; Subtypes (p. 339)

9. What are the three essential diagnostic features of anorexia nervosa?

   A. Persistently low self-confidence, intense fear of becoming fat, and disturbance in motivation.
   B. Low self-esteem, disturbance in self-perceived weight or shape, and persistent energy restriction.
   C. Restricted affect, disturbance in motivation, and low calorie intake.
   D. Persistent restriction of energy intake, intense fear of becoming fat, and disturbance in self-perceived weight or shape.
   E. Persistent lack of weight gain, disturbance in motivation, and restricted affect.

Correct Answer: D. Persistent restriction of energy intake, intense fear of becoming fat, and disturbance in self-perceived weight or shape.

Explanation: There are three essential features of anorexia nervosa: persistent energy intake restriction; intense fear of gaining weight or of becoming fat, or persistent behavior that interferes with weight gain; and a disturbance in self-perceived weight or shape.

9—Anorexia Nervosa / Diagnostic Features (pp. 239–240)

10. What laboratory abnormalities are commonly found in individuals with anorexia nervosa?

    A. Elevated blood urea nitrogen (BUN); low triiodothyronine (T_3); hyperadrenocorticism; low serum estrogen (females) or testosterone (males); bradycardia; low bone mineral density.
    B. Low BUN; hypercholesterolemia; high thyroxine (T_4); hypoadrenocorticism; short QTc; low bone mineral density.
    C. Blast cells; thrombocytosis; hyperphosphatemia; hypoamylasemia; high serum estrogen (females) or testosterone (males).
    D. Hyperzincemia; hypermagnesemia; hyperchloremia; hyperkalemia.
    E. C and D.

Correct Answer: A. Elevated blood urea nitrogen (BUN); low triiodothyronine (T_3); hyperadrenocorticism; low serum estrogen (females) or testosterone (males); bradycardia; low bone mineral density.

Explanation: Individuals with anorexia nervosa may have dehydration, reflected by elevated BUN levels. They may be cachectic and semistarved, reflected in other abnormal laboratory indices such as hypozincemia and hypophosphatemia. Purging, vomiting, and use of laxatives may lead to metabolic alkalosis, hypochloremia, and hypokalemia.

10—Anorexia Nervosa / Diagnostic Markers (pp. 342–343)

11. A 27-year-old graduate student has a 10-year history of anorexia nervosa. Her boyfriend is quite concerned because she has extreme fears related to cleanliness. She washes her hands more than 12 times a day and is excessively worried about contamination. What would be the best decision by the mental health professional at this point regarding these symptoms?

    A. Assume that the patient's obsessive-compulsive symptoms are related to her anorexia nervosa.
    B. Further evaluate the obsessive-compulsive features, because if they are not related to anorexia nervosa, a new diagnosis of obsessive-compulsive disorder might be warranted.
    C. Ask the patient to wait 1 year and see how this evolves.

D. Make a diagnosis of body dysmorphic disorder.

E. Refer the patient for a colonoscopy.

Correct Answer: B. Further evaluate the obsessive-compulsive features, because if they are not related to anorexia nervosa, a new diagnosis of obsessive-compulsive disorder might be warranted.

Explanation: Obsessive-compulsive features, both related and unrelated to food, are often prominent in anorexia nervosa. Most individuals with anorexia nervosa are preoccupied with thoughts of food. Some collect recipes or hoard food. Observations of behaviors associated with other forms of starvation suggest that obsessions and compulsions related to food may be exacerbated by undernutrition. When individuals with anorexia nervosa exhibit obsessions and compulsions that are not related to food, body shape, or weight, an additional diagnosis of obsessive-compulsive disorder may be warranted.

11—Anorexia Nervosa / Associated Features Supporting Diagnosis (p. 341)

12. What are the three essential diagnostic features of bulimia nervosa?

   A. Recurrent episodes of binge eating; recurrent inappropriate compensatory behaviors to prevent weight gain; self-evaluation that is unduly influenced by body shape and weight.
   B. Recurrent restriction of food; self-evaluation that is unduly influenced by body shape and weight; mood instability.
   C. Delusions regarding body habitus; obsessional focus on food; recurrent purging.
   D. Hypomanic symptoms for 1 month; mood instability; self-evaluation that is unduly influenced by body shape and weight.
   E. Self-evaluation that is unduly influenced by body shape and weight; history of anorexia nervosa; recurrent inappropriate compensatory behaviors to gain weight.

Correct Answer: A. Recurrent episodes of binge eating; recurrent inappropriate compensatory behaviors to prevent weight gain; self-evaluation that is unduly influenced by body shape and weight.

Explanation: There are three essential features of bulimia nervosa: recurrent episodes of binge eating, recurrent inappropriate compensatory behaviors to prevent weight gain, and self-evaluation that is unduly influenced by body shape and weight. To qualify for the diagnosis, the binge eating and inappropriate compensatory behaviors must occur, on average, at least once per week for 3 months. An "episode of binge eating" is defined as eating, in a discrete period of time, an amount of food that is definitely larger than most individuals would eat in a similar period of time under similar circumstances.

12—Bulimia Nervosa / Diagnostic Features (pp. 345–347)

13. What are the subtypes of bulimia nervosa?

   A. Restrictive.
   B. Purging.
   C. Restrictive and purging.
   D. None.
   E. With normal weight/abnormal weight.

Correct Answer: D. None.

Explanation: There are no subtypes for bulimia nervosa in DSM-5.

13—Bulimia Nervosa / diagnostic criteria (p. 345)

14. What minimum average frequency of binge eating is required to qualify for a diagnosis of binge-eating disorder?

   A. At least once a week for 3 months.
   B. At least twice a week for 3 months.
   C. At least once a week for 6 months.
   D. At least twice a week for 6 months.
   E. None of the above.

Correct Answer: A. At least once a week for 3 months.

Explanation: The essential feature of binge-eating disorder is recurrent episodes of binge eating that must occur, on average, at least once per week for 3 months. An "episode of binge eating" is defined as eating, in a discrete period of time, an amount of food that is definitely larger than most people would eat in a similar period of time under similar circumstances.

14—Binge-Eating Disorder / Diagnostic Features (pp. 350–351)